MEDICINE AND ART

Alan EH Emery and
Marcia LH Emery

Foreword by
Sir John Hanson

Dedicated to the memory of

Robert Platt,
Baron Platt of Grindleford
(1900–1978)

A renowned physician and lover of the arts

MEDICINE AND ART

Alan EH Emery and
Marcia LH Emery

Foreword by
Sir John Hanson

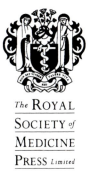

The ROYAL
SOCIETY *of*
MEDICINE
PRESS *Limited*

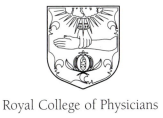

Royal College of Physicians

Published by the Royal Society of Medicine Press Ltd
in association with the Royal College of Physicians, London
©2003 Royal Society of Medicine Press Ltd
Reprinted 2004, 2006
1 Wimpole Street, London W1G 0AE, UK
207 E Westminster Road, Lake Forest, IL 60045, USA
www.rsmpress.co.uk

British Library Cataloguing in Publication Data
A catalogue record for this book is available from the British Library

ISBN 1-85315-501-2

Typeset by Phoenix Photosetting, Chatham, Kent, UK
Printed in Spain by T.G. Hostench, S.A.

CONTENTS

FOREWORD

"There really is no such thing as Art" wrote E.H. Gombrich, in the introduction to his monumental *The Story of Art* – "There are only artists". I suspect that Alan and Marcia Emery, joint authors of this beautifully rendered and revelatory book, might equally wish to make the same point about Medicine, which can never exist independently of the doctors. The headline, to be sure, is both Art and Medicine. But the revelation unfolded beneath it is a story as old as civilisation itself – the history of medicine if you will, but more revealingly, as the authors see it, a tale of healers and would-be healers in cultures and societies across measured time and across the globe.

The book is a classic, the typeface august, the illustrations selected with precision, the research meticulous, the volume published under both the imprint of The Royal Society of Medicine and the aegis of The Royal College of Physicians. It draws its material in a broad and spectacular sweep from the Pharoahs of Egypt and the veda of ancient India through the classical civilisation of the Mediterranean via European values to the present day. But the dramatic scale of the enterprise is moderated through a cool prose that is as limpid as it is laconic. The scientist authors eschew overstatement. The plot is uncovered perhaps more in the pictures than the text as the role of doctors, in their communities, shifts subtly but visibly through the centuries. The changes in the relationship between physician and patient reflect developments in the understanding and practice of medicine itself.

The work of the healer in early medicine is set in myth and magic and places the physician firmly at centre stage. It begins as his (usually his rather than her) story. We know relatively less about early patients. Were they actually healed? Were their would-be healers doctors or witch-doctors? Or must our growing understanding of traditional medicine systems cause us to rephrase that question? Does the dividing line between scientific and pre-scientific medicine grow justifiably dimmer? The sequence of more than fifty luminous plates provide a route map that throws into relief the twists and turns along the way. The doctor is seen no longer to stand alone, nurses and ancillaries appear alongside. Norman Rockwell's evocative family doctor is finally – after so long a period in which he could identify much but cure little – armed with modern instruments, technology and antibiotics. But now it is the patient who moves to centre stage. It is no longer just the doctor's tale.

Joint authorship always raises the question, as it does in this case: where does Alan Emery end and Marcia Emery begin? We do not, I think, need to know. Between them they marshal a distinguished research background and a profound knowledge of medicine and its taxonomy. In this College, where Alan's Fellowship association goes back to the mid-1980s – and his artistic talent is almost as well known as his work on neuromuscular diseases – we have been aware of *Medicine and Art* in gestation for almost five years. Its vision is integrated, rich and complex. The artist and the scientist make the same homage to crucial detail, no two cultures here. The wait has been amply rewarded.

Sir John Hanson
Green College, Oxford 2002

ACKNOWLEDGEMENTS

We should like to express our appreciation to all the individuals and galleries who gave us permission to reproduce works of art. Several are living artists and among these we should particularly like to thank Sir Roy Calne and Sergei Chepik and his wife Marie-Aude Albert.

There are however many other individuals who gave us much useful advice and help whom we should like to thank personally. They include William Schupbach, Curator of the Iconographic Collection of the Wellcome Library; Dr Nigel Allan, Curator of Oriental Manuscripts of the Wellcome Library; Julia Beckwith of the Royal College of Physicians Library, London; A.W. Potter, Research Assistant, Library of the Royal Academy; Susannah Gilbert, Collections Assistant, Wolverhampton Art Gallery; Clara Young, Heritage Officer, Arts, Dundee; Rhian Harris, Coram Foundling Museum, London; Mr William Dinning; Professor Michel Fardeau, La Salpêtrière; and Dr Peter Watkins, Editor of *Clinical Medicine* (Journal of the Royal College of Physicians of London) who first encouraged us to undertake the project and has given permission to reproduce several essays previously published in the journal (numbers, 9, 12, 13, 15, 18, 19, 22, 23, 30, 33, 35, 36, 40, 43, and 44).

Most importantly we are especially grateful for the help of Mr Bill Hopkins and his staff of the Department of Medical Illustration of the University of Edinburgh, and to Mr Peter Richardson, Managing Director and Ms Gabrielle Lowis of the Royal Society of Medicine Press for their continued support and encouragement. Finally we are most grateful to the Warden, Sir John Hanson, and Fellows of Green College, Oxford, for providing facilities for researching and writing the book.

Oxford, 2002

INTRODUCTION

The relationship between medicine and art has attracted much interest from writers and commentators over the years, and has been considered from various points of view. The most obvious is the depiction of various medical conditions in paintings[1,2] and we have listed many such examples in the Appendix. Another approach has been to analyse the effects medical conditions may have on an artist's creativity.[3,4] Interest has centred for example on physical disabilities such as Renoir's rheumatoid arthritis,[5] and the effects of eye disease,[6,7] including colour blindness[8] and of course Monet's cataracts.[9] The effects of mental illness[10–12] on the work of professional artists have also been considered since they may help our understanding of the neuropathology of these diseases, for example cases of dementia[13,14] and encephalitis.[15] The revealing effects of multiple sclerosis have been described in detail by Peter MacKarell, an English artist who suffered from the disease in the last eight years or so of his life.[16] Many celebrated artists have also become alcoholic with effects on their creativity.[17] Furthermore, illness may not only affect *how* an artist paints but also *what* he paints. For example, R.B. Kitaj (b. 1932), began walking on his doctor's advice to take more exercise after suffering a severe heart attack; this in due course led him to a new range of subjects.[18]

Yet another aspect of the topic is consideration of diagnostic techniques and medical treatment in works of art.[19] Here we consider works of art which reflect the physician's role in society and the relationship between doctor and patient. These are sometimes different in different societies and have clearly changed over time. We have attempted to select work which we feel best illustrates these points and to give an international perspective. This is particularly relevant today in view of changing attitudes to the profession, at least in part due to society's increasing expectations.

The illustrations have been mainly arranged in the chronological order in which they were created but sometimes to reflect noteworthy events in the history of medicine. For example the introduction of smallpox vaccination by Jenner in 1798 and of the stethoscope by Laënnec in 1816 were depicted by artists some time after the events.

In a book of this size we have only been able to include a fraction of all the works on the subject. Our selection has therefore been somewhat eclectic and much influenced by our own personal preferences. What did become very clear to us was that the works of art can often reflect quite revealingly the role of the physician in society. Though Thomas Carlyle was referring to the written word, his thoughts could equally apply to works of 'medicine and art':

What is all knowledge but recorded experience

Or as John Berger in his *Ways of Seeing* has written more recently:[20]

No other kind of relic or text from the past can offer such a direct testimony about the world which surrounded other people at other times. In this respect images are more precise and richer than literature. To say this is not to deny the expressive or imaginative quality of art, treating it as mere documentary evidence; the more imaginative the work, the more profoundly it allows us to share the artist's experience of the visible.

References

1. Kunze J, Nippert I. *Genetics and malformations in art.* Berlin: Grosse Verlag, 1986.
2. Enderle A, Meyerhöfer D, Unverfehrt G. *Small people – great art.* Hamm: Artcolor Verlag, 1994.
3. Sandblom P. *Creativity and disease.* New York, London: Marion Boyars, 1992.

4. Emery AEH. Medicine, artists and their art. *J Roy Coll Phys Lond 1997*; **31**: 450–455.

5. Boonen A, van de Rest J, Dequeker J, van der Linden S. How Renoir coped with rheumatoid arthritis. *BMJ* 1997; **315**: 1704–1708.

6. Trevor-Roper P. *The world through blunted sight*. New revised edition. London: Allen Lane, Penguin Press, 1988.

7. Elliott DB, Skaff A. Vision of the famous: the artist's eye. *Ophthal Physiol Opt* 1993; **13**: 82–90.

8. Ravin JG, Anderson N, Lanthony P. An artist with a color vision defect: Charles Meryon. *Survey of Ophthalmol* 1995; **39**: 403–408.

9. Ravin JG. Monet's cataracts. *JAMA* 1985; **254**: 394–399

10. Critchley EMR. *Hallucinations and their impact on art*. Preston: Carnegie Press, 1987.

11. MacGregor JM. *The discovery of the art of the insane*. Princeton, New Jersey: Princeton University Press, 1989.

12. Gilman SL. *Disease and representation: images of illness from madness to AIDS*. Ithaca, New York: Cornell University Press, 1994.

13. Espinel CH. De Kooning's late colours and forms: dementia, creativity, and the healing power of art. *Lancet* 1996; **347**, 1096–1098.

14. Crutch SJ, Isaacs R, Rossor MN. Some workmen can blame their tools: artistic change in an individual with Alzheimer's disease. *Lancet 2001*; **357**: 2129–2133.

15. Stanhope N, Kopelman MD. Art and memory: a 7-year follow-up of herpes encephalitis in a professional artist. *Neurocase 2000*; **6**: 99–110.

16. MacKarell P. *Depictions of an odyssey*. Corsham, Wilts: National Society for Education in Art and Design (NSEAD), 1990.

17. Beveridge A, Yorston G. I drink, therefore I am: alcohol and creativity. *J Roy Soc Med* 1999; **92**: 646–648.

18. Delamothe T. Kitaj's 'heart attack'. *BMJ* 1993; **307**: 1617.

19. Emery AEH, Emery MLH. Medicine and art: diagnosis and medical treatment. *Proc Roy Coll Phys Edin* 1992; **22**: 519–542.

20. Berger J. *Ways of seeing*. London: BBC and Penguin, 1972.

The Plates

1

Early medicine

The earliest documented physician of note was Imhotep the royal chamberlain to the Egyptian King Ketjerkhet (Djoser) of the Third Dynasty (c 2686–2613 BC). He treated the King and over the following millennia he was worshipped as the life-giving son of the god Ptah. After visiting Egypt before the first World War and studying the antiquities, William Osler is quoted as concluding that Imhotep was 'the first figure of a physician to stand out clearly from the mists of antiquity'. Later in the Ptolemaic Period the ancient Greeks identified him with Asclepius (or Asklepios), their god of medicine, and later the Romans with their healing god of mythology (Aesculapius).

But these gods reflected the then current mythical explanations for illness. The first individual to be credited with a rational approach to disease was Hippocrates (c 460–370 BC), a Greek physician born on the Island of Cos, who studied medicine at Cos, Ionia, Egypt and Asia. He gathered together all he considered sound in medical practice up until his time and is credited with having written over 70 works on the subject. Though there is some doubt about the precise authorship of all these works, he is generally acknowledged as the real father of modern medicine. For a time the faith healing tradition of Asclepius and the more rational Hippocratic medicine continued side by side in Greece. According to E.D. Phillips [in his *Aspects of Greek Medicine* (Croom Helm, 1987)]

> 'It may be guessed that when physicians of the kind that we may with some reservations call secular refused to treat the incurably sick, they were in effect entrusting them to the unexplained powers of Asclepius, as revealed by his priests…'

Hippocrates however separated medicine from mythology and philosophy, and the many aphorisms attributed to him contain much common sense: 'Life is short but the Art is Long'. He was the first to record case histories, and to base medical practice on bedside observation and he provided doctors with ethical and moral standards embodied in the Hippocratic Oath. He travelled and taught far and wide and was consulted by the rich and famous of the time including King Perdiccas of Macedon and Ataxerxes of Persia.

Over time there have been many impressions, mainly in sculpture, of Hippocrates' appearance. All of these are now believed to be imaginative with but one exception. It seems that the most reliable depiction is on Roman coins of the first century AD from the Island of Cos bearing the name Hippocrates. This appearance resembles that of a Roman copy of a Greek statue found near Ostia in 1940. The reverse side of the coin shows the serpent-entwined staff of Asclepius which subsequently became included in the coat of arms of many medical societies and associations, including the logo of the World Health Organisation.

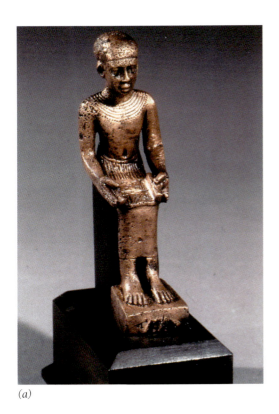

(a)

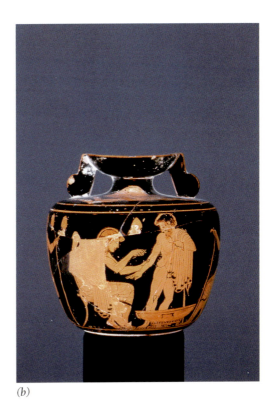

(b)

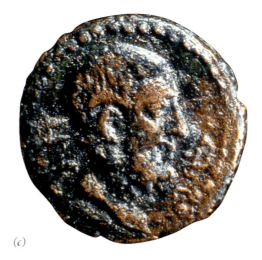

(c)

(a) Typical copper alloy statue of Imhotep, deified long after his death. He is seated with a papyrus roll on his knee (26th Dynasty). (©The British Museum); (b) Perfume vessel of the time of Hippocrates, 5 century BC, with decorations attributed to the Painter of the Clinic, showing physician treating the patient's arm, presumably after having bled him. (The Louvre, Paris. © Photo RMN – Hervé Lewandowski); (c) Roman coin showing Hippocrates' head from 1 century AD from the island of Cos (©The British Museum).

2

An Ayurvedic Practitioner Taking the Pulse (Delhi, c 1830)

artist unknown

The Vedas are a compilation of Hindu texts dating from around 1000 BC and apart from being religious they also contain much medical instruction. From around 500 BC further commentaries also became incorporated in so-called 'Ayurvedic' medicine with practical advice on all aspects of life, the term Ayurvedic being derived from the Sanskrit, meaning knowledge (*veda*) for longevity (*ayus*). Prevention of disease is important, with an emphasis on personal hygiene and with moderation in all things, including food, exercise, sex and dosage of medicines. The pharmacopoeia of traditional Ayurvedic medicine includes a vast variety of substances of plant, animal and mineral origin. The Indian plant *Rauwolfia serpentina*, or snake root, from which the alkaloid reserpine was derived, was introduced into Western medicine in the 1950s for the treatment of hypertension, though is now superseded by other compounds with fewer side-effects.

Over time various diagnostic techniques became incorporated, beginning with urine examination and pulse taking and subsequently consideration of the patient's tongue, eyes, skin and general appearance, and nowadays a comprehensive examination. Later there were influences from Islamic and Western medicine but traditional Indian medicine remains essentially holistic. According to a description given by the 5th century Chinese pilgrim Fa Hsien, present-day Patna in India was the site of probably the world's first organised hospital-based health care system.

The practitioner as well as the apprentice student in Ayurvedic medicine is expected to conform to the highest standards in his professional and personal life, including his dress and behaviour. Even today Ayurvedic medicine is widely practised in India, especially in the countryside, often alongside Western medicine. It enjoys State support and there are Ayurvedic colleges and hospitals all over India. In 1985 there were around 100 officially accredited Ayurvedic colleges, many attached to universities and clinics. Apart from Ayurveda, students receive some basic education in Western medicine as well as family planning and public health.

In this Indian watercolour painting from the early part of the 19th century, an Ayurvedic practitioner is examining a patient and taking his pulse, though the artist has failed to show the doctor's fingers in the correct position for taking the radial pulse. The small circular objects may have been for cupping or more likely were containers for various traditional medicines. There is also a lacquered box for surgical instruments which would have been largely used at the time for venesection. There is also a head-rest in the foreground. The dress of the practitioner and patient as well as tree foliage in the background indicate a location in northern India.

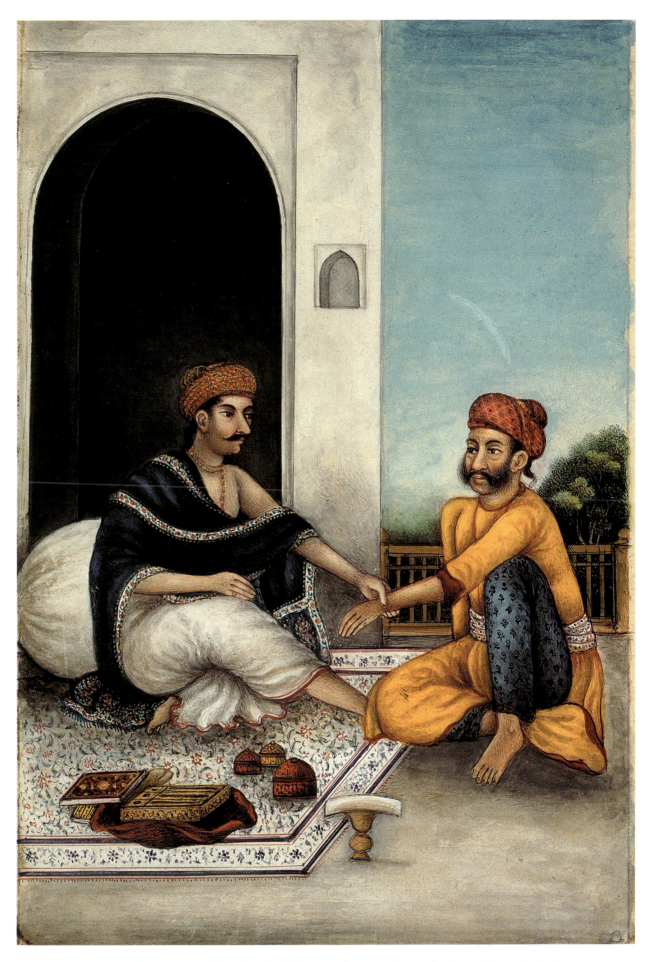

An Ayurvedic Practitioner Taking the Pulse (Delhi, c 1830), artist unknown (Wellcome Library, London).

3

Medical Painting from Central Tibet (1800–1899)

Buddhism was founded by Prince Gautama (the Buddha or the 'Enlightened One', 563–483 BC) and from its inception emphasised peace of mind by contemplation and abandonment of desire. As the Buddha's followers increased over the years, Buddhist monks in their monasteries became increasingly involved in caring for the sick, at first among their fellow brethren, but later in the community at large. Some of the most beautifully illustrated works concerning Buddhist traditions of medicine are found in certain Tibetan texts.

The Tibetan Medical Institute is now based in Dharamsala in North India. Here Tibetan doctors receive their education for a minimum of seven years which includes both theoretical and practical training. Without going into details, the essentials of Tibetan medicine involve changes in dietary habits, meditation and rest, prescription of various herbal remedies and physical treatment which may included moxa (burning of small pellets of material at points on the skin), blood-letting, mild emetics and purgation, massage and acupuncture. Some of these measures are shown in the accompanying illustration taken from a medical painting from Central Tibet (1800–1899).

The Tibetan Buddhist tradition of medicine, as also in Chinese and Indian traditional medicine, is essentially holistic with an emphasis on natural remedies and techniques. This is often nowadays referred to as alternative or complementary medicine. It has increased in popularity in the West in recent years no doubt because patients may expect more from, and therefore in some cases are likely to be more disappointed by, modern scientifically-based medicine. In recent years the Royal Society of Medicine has encouraged 'bridge building' between conventional and alternative approaches to treatment.

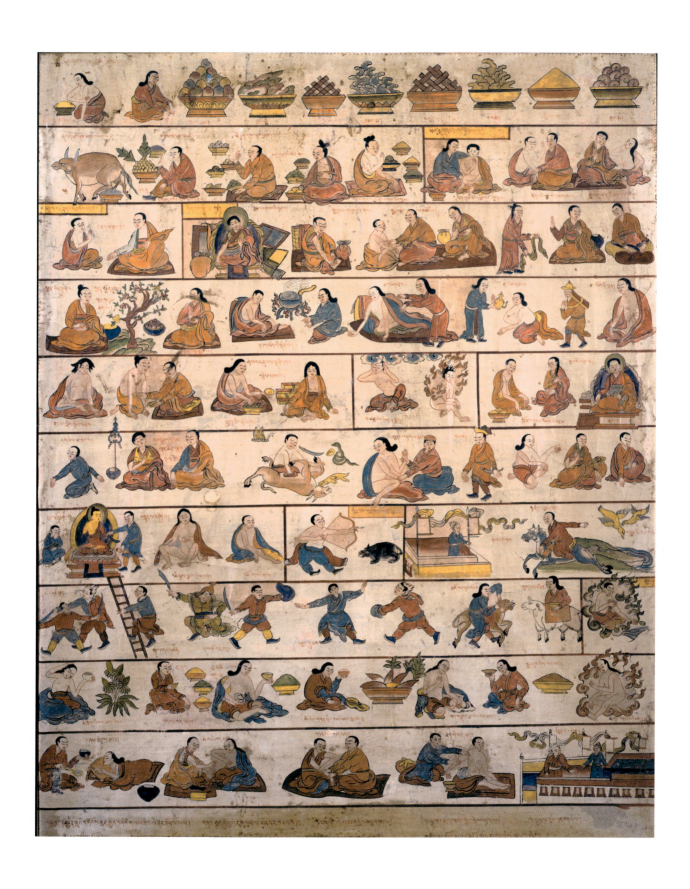

Medical Painting from Central Tibet (1800–1899). Ground mineral pigment on cotton (Courtesy of the Collection of Shelley & Donald Rubin; www.himalyanart.org).

4

Physician taking a Patient's Pulse in a Persian Garden (17th century) from the cover of a copy of Avicenna's *Canon of Medicine*

Early medical teaching was most notably dominated by Galen (AD 129–c 216) who was born in Pergamon, now Bergama in Turkey. He was not only a fine clinician, but also became renowned for his anatomical knowledge though this was based on the dissection of animals but not humans. He is credited with some 350 works, with no less than 16 books on the pulse alone. Early Greek medical teaching, especially that of Galen, was much appreciated by an emerging Islam. These teachings were assimilated and elaborated upon particularly by Abu al-Husain ibn Abdallah ibn Sina, known in the West as Avicenna (AD 980–1037), who was born in Persia and travelled widely in the region. His *Canon of Medicine (Al-Qanun)* was to have considerable influence throughout the Middle Ages, and was widely used both in the Islamic world as well as in Latin translation in the West. It was in fact mentioned by Geoffrey Chaucer in the Prologue to his *Canterbury Tales*. It was highly regarded as an authoritative, comprehensive, well-organised and systematic text. It was a vast compendium of medical knowledge consisting of five books which dealt with the presumed causes of illness, details of specific diseases and treatment. This illustration, of Safavid Persian lacquer work of the 17th century, is one of two papier mâché boards which bound an exemplar of Avicenna's *Canon*. It shows a physician taking the pulse of a lady while attendants prepare various medications. It refers to an incident when a physician, taking a young lady's pulse in order to diagnose her condition, mentions a particular young man's name. On hearing his name, the patient's pulse quickens and the physician diagnoses 'love-sickness'.

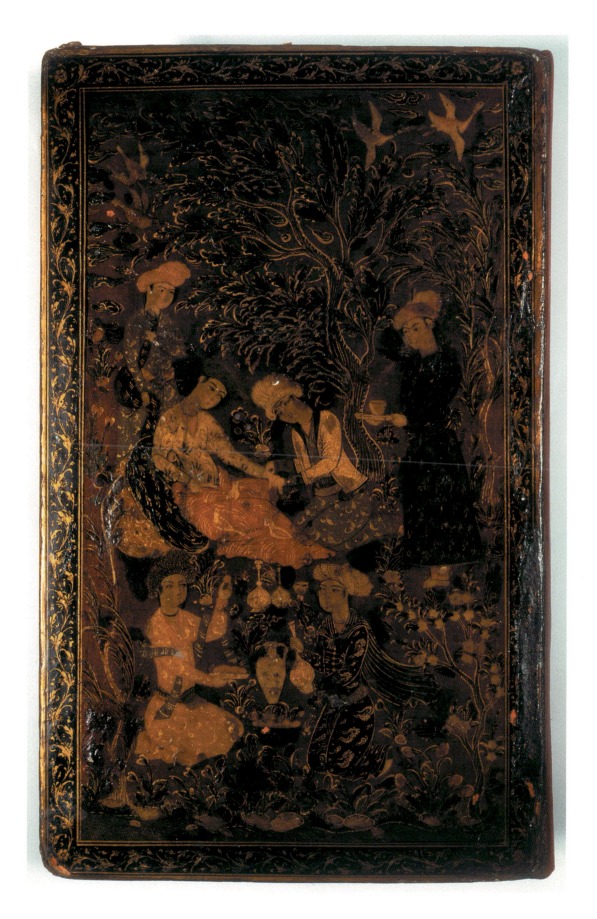

Physician Taking a Patient's Pulse in a Persian Garden (17th century). From the cover of a copy of Avicenna's *Canon of Medicine* (Wellcome Library, London).

5

Hippocrates Medicating a Patient
(13th century) from *De regimine acutorum*

This 13th century miniature is one of the very earliest depictions in Britain of a medical consultation. It is at the beginning of the treatise *De regimine acutorum* and purports to show Hippocrates treating a patient. But since no such portrait of Hippocrates existed at the time, he is shown merely as a contemporary university doctor of medicine in his traditional gown and cap, thus emphasising his authoritative status. It may be the patient was suffering from a fever, which Hippocrates emphasised was the mark of an acute illness. At the time this was likely to be attributed to the 'ague', a general term for a febrile illness which included malaria, the last locally acquired case of which occurred in the English Fenland some 70 years ago. The so-called 'English sweating sickness', possibly a severe viral infection, would later also have been a common concern of the practitioner. Here the physician appears to be administering a liquid from a shallow dish, since the actual text is much concerned with the virtues of various liquid preparations which included wine and particularly ptisan or barley water. The third person by the bedside may have been an assistant or apprentice.

At the time several universities had been founded, beginning with Salerno in the 11th century and followed by Paris (1110), Bologna (1158), Oxford (1167), Montpellier (1181), Cambridge (1209) and Padua (1222), where medical training was initially informal but later became organised into official faculties. Most practitioners would have trained in one of these centres or been apprenticed to someone who had been. Excluding barber-surgeons, it has been estimated that there were fewer than 1000 active practitioners in England in the 13th century and their authority would have been unchallenged as seems to be the case in this illustration.

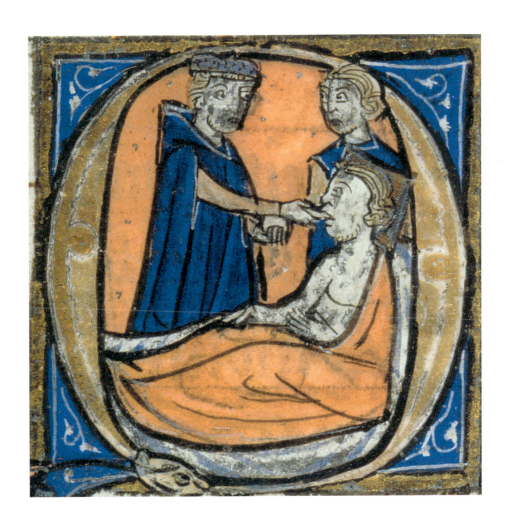

Hippocrates Medicating a Patient (13th century) from *De regimine acutorum* (The British Library, Harley MS 3140, f. 39).

6

St Humility Healing a Sick Nun (c 1341)

by Pietro Lorenzetti

Medical care, in the West, until relatively recently was almost entirely under the patronage of the Christian Church. The clergy and monks were often responsible for ministering to the sick, for after all they were usually the only educated people able to read and write, and therefore familiar with medical practices elsewhere. Nursing care was provided by nuns who were members of religious orders, notably Daughters of Charity founded by Vincent de Paul. Though divine considerations were pre-eminent, so that sickness was viewed as the result of sin and recovery due to the intervention of Providence, a temporal approach developed with increasing emphasis on the care and shelter of the sick. This painting illustrates the role of the Church in the care of the sick.

St Humility (1226–1310) came from an aristocratic family in Faenza in Northern Italy. After she had married for nine years, with her husband's approval, she entered a convent. Eventually she became an abbess and later founded a convent of her own order near Florence. She became sanctified after her death, and by tradition is depicted with a lambskin on top of her order's head-dress to emphasise her humility and gentleness. Here she is in a convent ministering to a sick nun who is sitting up in bed. But in the adjoining room a physician gestures his helplessness at the sight of a blood-filled vessel from the patient. Perhaps this was a case of tuberculosis.

The artist Pietro Lorenzetti (active 1320–1348) and his brother Ambrogio were both Sienese painters and much influenced by Giotto (c 1266–1337) who is credited with being the earliest Renaissance painter. Little is known of the brothers' lives except that both died in 1348 from the Black Death which ravaged Northern Italy with particular severity and killed off most of the artists of the time.

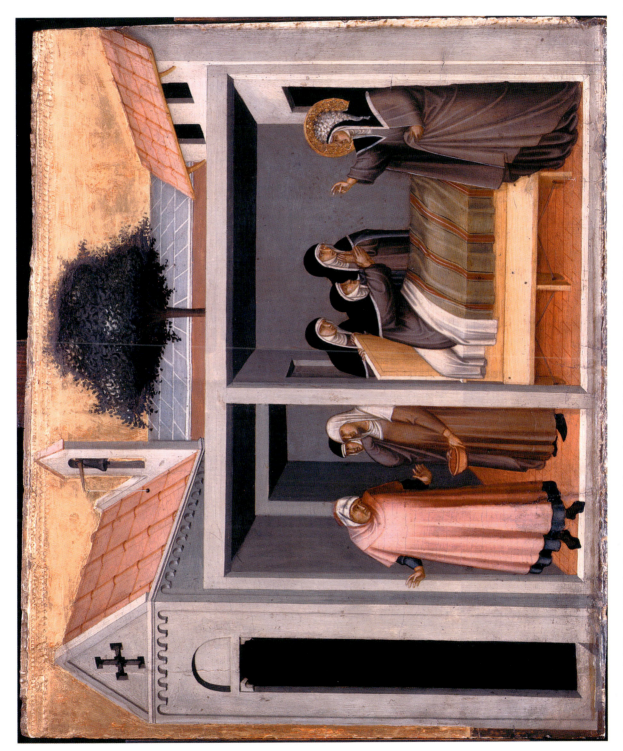

7

Illustration from a French translation of *De Proprietatibus Rerum* (late 15th century)

by Bartholomew Anglicus

Until the introduction of printing in the mid-15th century, authors depended on the manual transcription and illustration of their work in manuscripts. Many of these in fact became works of art in their own right. Bartholomew Anglicus, or the Englishman (active 1230–1250), was an English-born Franciscan friar who studied in Paris where he eventually became a famous Professor of Theology. One chronicler of the time referred to him as 'a great clerk who read through the whole Bible in lectures at Paris'. He was later sent to Saxony in 1231 to help organise a branch of the order.

His great work *De Proprietatibus Rerum* was a compilation of 19 books on various aspects of human knowledge and was a source of common information throughout the Middle Ages. It was first printed in Basle about 1470 and went through 14 or more editions before 1500, and was translated from the Latin into various languages including French, English and Spanish. It is believed that Shakespeare may well have been acquainted with the work.

In this beautiful illustration taken from a late 15th century French translation of the manuscript, on the left a physician is ministering to his sick patient. He holds up and inspects a flask of the patient's urine. Uroscopy was then the most important aspect of the investigation of a patient, upon which a diagnosis and treatment were based. He points to the apothecary's shop where medicinal products are being carefully weighed. In an attempt to avoid fraudulent weights and measures, inspections of these establishments began to take place as early as the 14th century. We can also recognise the various apothecary's jars, drawers for preserving vegetable products, and a cask for storing herbs, roots, and so on.

The illustration could be interpreted as the physician and the apothecary having separate roles. But in fact the two roles were often undertaken by the same individual until very much later.

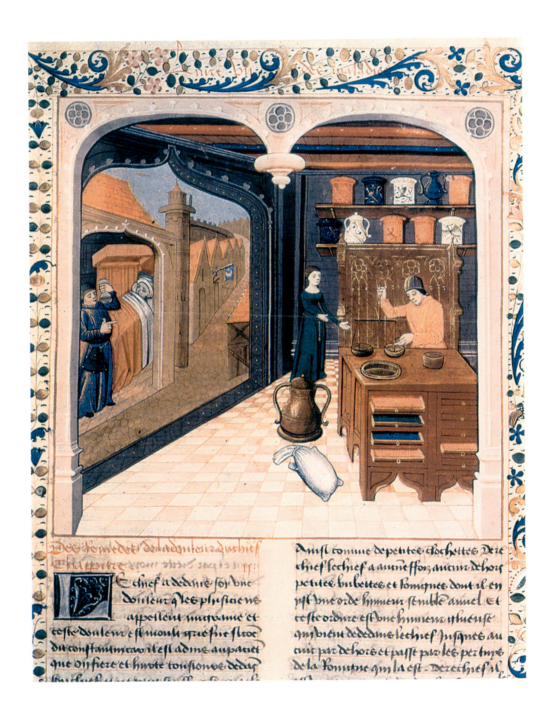

Illustration from a French translation of De Proprietatibus Rerum (late 15th century) by Bartholomew Anglicus (Cliché Bibliothèque nationale de France, Paris).

8

St Francis Healing the Leper (c 1630) by Giovanni Battista Crespi (called Il Cerano)

In the early history of the Christian Church disease and sickness, like all other evils, were often regarded as a consequence of sin and recovery was interpreted as the result of divine intervention. But at the same time the Church respected the powers of secular healing and, as in Greek and Roman times, religious and secular attitudes often co-existed. In fact Christianity gave rise to new centres of religious healing, both spiritual and physical, often based on monasteries where religious communities would care for the sick. In England these included for example St Bartholomew's Hospital and St Thomas' Hospital, both founded in the early 12th century. Though originally of a religious nature these establishments, particularly following the Reformation, later became staffed more by trained surgeons and physicians. This painting clearly indicated that in 17th century Italy religious establishments continued to play a major role in the care of the sick.

The artist, Giovanni Battista Crespi (c 1575–1632), also know as Il Cerano, was not only a painter but also an engraver, sculptor, architect and writer. He spent almost all his life working in Milan. Early in his career he was befriended by Cardinal Federico Borromeo, who became the painter's major patron. Most of Crespi's work in fact has a religious theme and includes many altarpieces and Church commissions. His work has been said to represent a transition between the so-called Mannerist style and the Baroque. The former followed the Renaissance from around 1520 to 1600 and was characterised by primacy of the human figure, which was often elongated and depicted in strained poses. It was essentially subjective and emotionally often created a feeling of ambiguity and discomfort. Some of these characteristics are evident in this painting. The pose of the leper indicates discomfort in his shoulder and the caring attention of St Francis and his attendant is all too clear. This scene recalls the healing of a leper by Christ Himself (Matt. 8: 1–4, Mark 1: 40–45, Luke 5: 12–16) and at the time of the painting observers would no doubt have considered such divine healing as a real possibility.

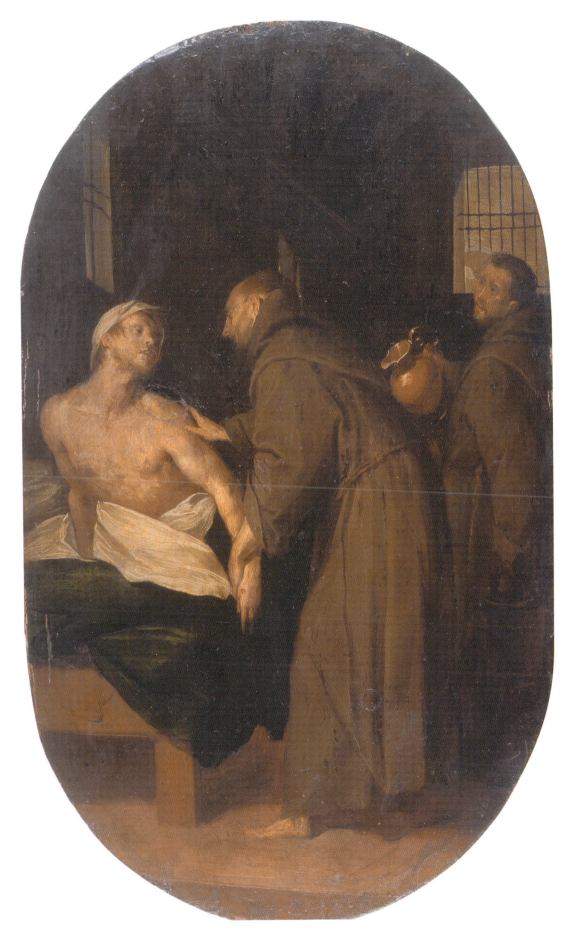

St Francis Healing the Leper (c 1630) by Giovanni Battista Crespi (called Il Cerano). Pinacoteca di Brera, Milan. (Under licence from Italian Ministry for Cultural Goods and Activities)

9

The Quack Doctor (1652)

by Gerrit Dou

The Oxford Dictionary defines a 'quack' as an ignorant pretender to medical knowledge who professes a skill or treatment. In bygone days quack doctors were much in evidence because there were in fact few effective treatments and no doubt the general public was also more gullible than nowadays. Certainly the subject attracted the attention of many artists in the past, including William Hogarth (1697–1764) in Britain and several Dutch genre painters of the 17th century, most notably Gerrit Dou (1613–1675) of Leiden. Dou was first apprenticed to his father, a glass engraver, then became associated with the young Rembrandt, though their styles and subjects diverged considerably in later life. In 1648 he became a founding member of the Leiden Guild of St Luke which emphasised the historical links between the physician and the painter. In this painting the artist has actually portrayed himself seated in a window looking at the viewer. Dou was much admired in his day and counted among his patrons Charles II of England, Queen Christina of Sweden and Archduke Leopold Wilhelm of Austria. But despite his international reputation he rarely left his native city. He remained a bachelor all his life and died in Leiden in 1675.

His work is characterised by meticulously crafted portraits, still-lifes and genre pieces, often quite small and for which as an aid he used a concave glass system of his own design. In this picture he depicts the quack selling potions under a Chinese umbrella. To enhance his credibility he is dressed in the academic robes associated at the time with a qualified physician. The gathering crowd depicts the varying responses to the quack's claims. The hunter seems convinced of the potion's value, but a housewife on the right seems more sceptical. Perhaps this is a love potion, and behind the hunter a young man appears to be attempting to convince his partner of its possible value. As one looks more closely at the painting it becomes clear that Dou is also concerned with other issues: the mother cleaning the baby's bottom is possibly a scatological commentary on the doctor's exalted claims, and could the little boy trying to catch a bird imply the elusiveness of trying to find an effective cure? As in all such genre paintings there is much more than a cursory glance would suggest.

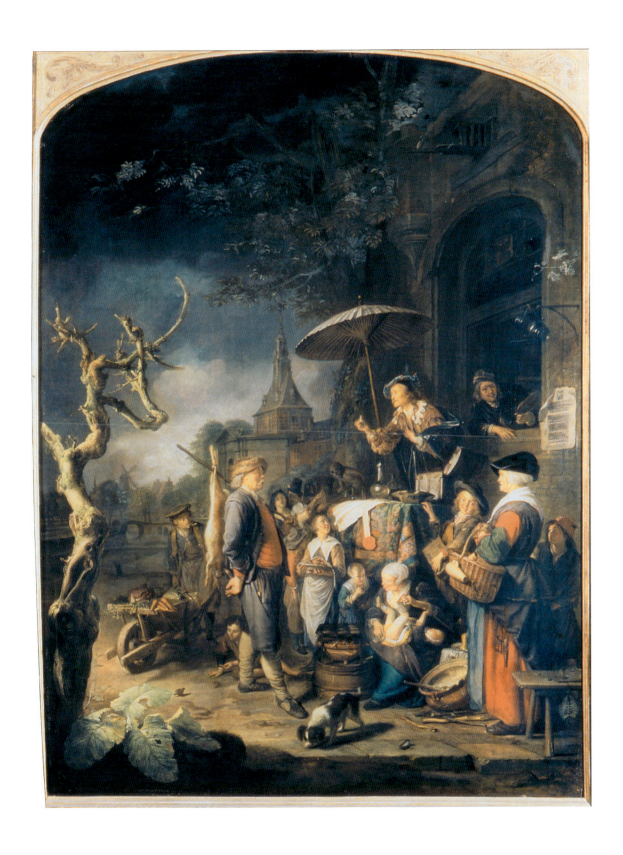

The Quack Doctor (1652) by Gerrit Dou (reproduced by kind permission of the Museum Boijmans Van Beuningen, Rotterdam).

10

The Village Doctor (c 1650)

by David Teniers the Younger

Until the eighteenth century the physician's diagnostic techniques consisted of little more than pulse taking and visual inspection of the urine or uroscopy. The latter was a survival from ancient times and had developed into a fine art, and from which the practitioner would make some profound diagnosis. Dr Thomas Willis (1621–1675) had discovered diabetes by noting the sweet taste of the urine, but as practised by uroscopists the technique was worthless. They were considered charlatans and in the eighteenth century were often referred to as 'pisse-prophets'. Some of these individuals however became enormously wealthy through the practice including a Theodore von Myersbach who, having purchased his medical degree in Germany, came to London in 1770 to proffer his diagnostic skill to the gullible.

It is quite likely however that some practitioners may have mistakenly believed that uroscopy could be a help in diagnosis and this may have been the case in this delightful and detailed painting of a rustic doctor. He is seen surrounded by the paraphernalia of his profession with a large flask of urine and several large reference tomes open on his table. The patient apprehensively considers the physician's reaction to his urine sample.

David Teniers the Younger (1610–1690) was a Flemish painter from Antwerp whose work was much appreciated at the time and in 1651 he was appointed Court Painter and Custodian of the Art Collection in Brussels. This work was painted around this time.

Many painters of the seventeenth and eighteenth centuries, particularly Dutch and Flemish artists, often ridiculed uroscopists with their pretentious, grave manner and flamboyant and theatrical dress. Teniers has painted a more sympathetic picture. However it seems likely the artist was not entirely convinced of the value of the practice because on the wall on the right is pinned an unflattering cartoon picture of a uroscopist.

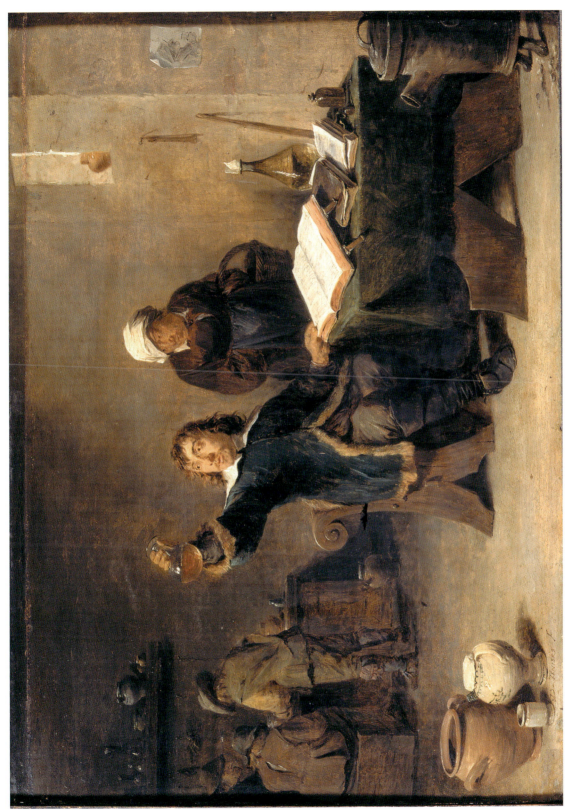

The Village Doctor (c 1650) by David Teniers the Younger (Musées royaux des Beaux-Arts de Belgique – Koninklijke Musea voor Schone Kunsten van België, Brussel).

11

The Physician (1653)

by Gerrit Dou

This painting, though the subject matter is the same as in the preceding work by Teniers, is more a vehicle for demonstrating the artist's talents. The textures of the doctor's garments and carpet thrown over his table, as well as the surfaces of the bronze dish used in bloodletting and the stoppered container, are all painted with great skill. A copy of Vesalius' *De Humani Corporis Fabrica* is included in the physician's possessions to add gravitas and the implication of learning. The painter Gerrit Dou (1613–1675) of Leiden worked on a small scale (this painting is less than 50 × 40 cm) with a surface of almost enamelled smoothness. Lighting has been used to emphasise the physician's facial expression. All is depicted with the artist's consummate skill. The painting can be appreciated not only as censure of the pretentious charlatan, but also as a work of art by a very talented artist.

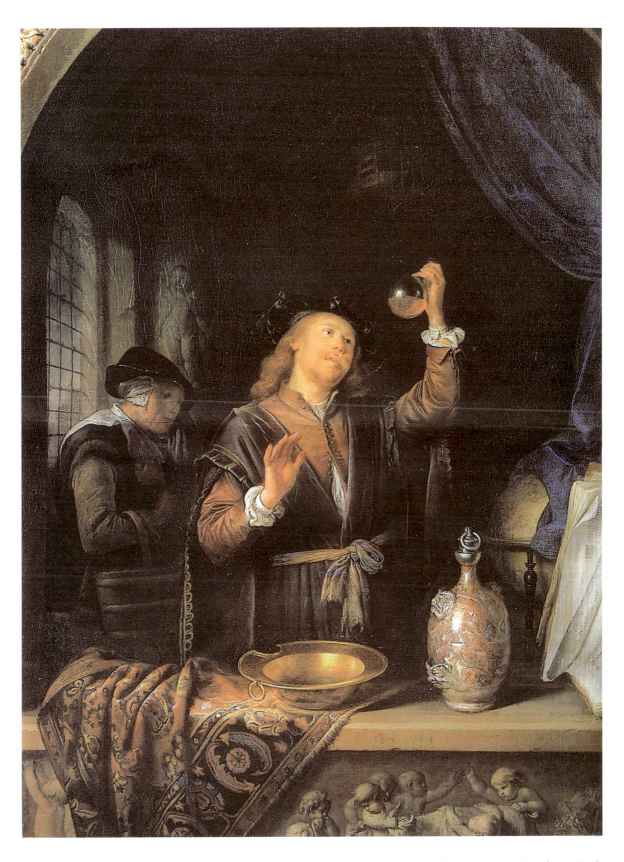

The Physician (1653) by Gerrit Dou (reproduced by kind permission of the Christchurch Gallery Te Puna o Waiwhetu, Heathcote Helmore bequest, 1965, New Zealand).

12

The Doctor's Visit (c 1663)

by Jan Steen

Jan Steen (1626–1679) was a prolific Dutch painter mainly of humorous subjects often depicting everyday tavern scenes or, as in this case, a doctor's visit. In the 17th century the physician's diagnostic tools were limited often to little more than an examination of the urine and pulse, as Steen demonstrates in this painting. However, as in many of these genre paintings of the time, the artist is not so much concerned with demonstrating a medical consultation as such, but more with social issues and morality.

Steen painted the subject of a doctor's visit at least 18 times. The patient is always a young lady whom the artist indicates by various symbols in the picture to be suffering from love-sickness, erotic melancholy or early pregnancy. In this case the attitude of the lady with her head leaning on her hand indicated at the time that she was a melancholic (her pet dog appears concerned and mimics her mood). Repressed and unrequited love were believed to be the cause. In fact the artist provides several clues in the painting which suggest this is the case of '*maladie d'amour*': the picture of a love scene (Venus and Adonis) on the back wall, the brazier with smouldering ribbon (at the time a folk custom for determining pregnancy), and the cupid-like young boy with his bow and arrows.

However the painter leaves the observer with several unresolved questions. Is the man poring over his papers in the back room her husband and is he unconcerned, perhaps neglecting his conjugal duty, or has he been cuckolded? Furthermore are the purse and keys hanging on the back of the chair an indication that she is also neglecting her own duties as a housewife? As in many of Steen's paintings we are left to reflect on matters of morality and conscience.

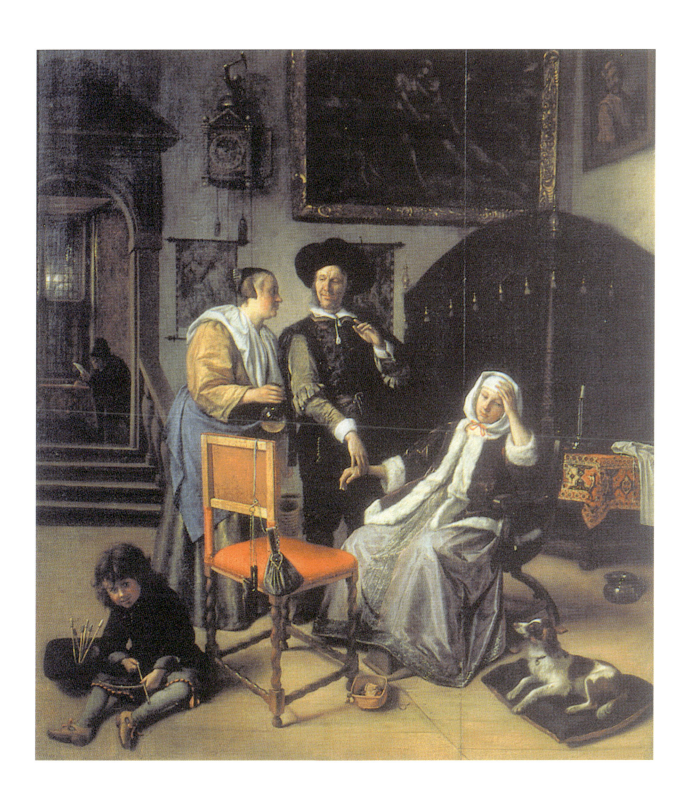

The Doctor's Visit (c 1663) by Jan Steen (courtesy of the Trustees of the V & A, London).

13

Marriage à la Mode: The Inspection (1743)
by William Hogarth

William Hogarth (1697–1764) commenting on his paintings and engravings of moral subjects wrote '… I have endeavoured to treat my subjects as a dramatic writer; my picture is my stage, and men and women are my players, who by means of certain actions and gestures are to exhibit a dumb show.' The first of these moral subjects was the series *The Harlot's Progress* (1731–2), followed by *The Rake's Progress* (1735), *Marriage à la Mode* (1743) and finally *The Election* (1754). Each is a detailed and critical commentary on behaviour and customs of the time in England in the 18th century.

This particular painting, *The Inspection*, belongs to the series *Marriage à la Mode*, which traces the disastrous marriage between an idle, supercilious and dissipated earl's son to a spoilt daughter of a rich merchant. Firstly there is *The Marriage Contract* when the marriage is arranged, secondly the *Tête à Tête (Breakfast Scene)* where the newly-weds are exhausted after an all-night card-party. The scene clearly indicates that their lifestyle has resulted in serious debt and the young nobleman's life of debauchery has resulted in his acquiring a venereal disease. In *The Inspection*, the nobleman visits a French quack doctor ('Mon' de la Pillule') for treatment. The remaining scenes (*The Toilette, Death of the Earl,* and *Death of the Countess*) chart the subsequent downfall of the couple.

As in all of Hogarth's moral series, there is much detail and research has revealed a great deal of its significance. The scene and surroundings represent a criticism of quackery in general: the grotesque appearance of the quack himself, the many objects and images referring to useless remedies. The model head with a pill in its mouth was often displayed outside an apothecary's shop in order to advertise his wares. The urinal represents the practice of uroscopy. The unicorn's horn was a highly-prized and expensive medieval remedy and supposed aphrodisiac. There is much more. The nobleman holds out a box of pills, the lid remaining on his seat, indicating the area for treatment. He is portrayed with a black spot on his neck, indicating venereal infection which appears in subsequent images in the series, including later his child by the countess.

Hogarth was very critical of the quack doctors of his time and the gullibility of many patients. His sympathy for the sick themselves however is beautifully illustrated in *The Pool of Bethesda* painted on the staircase of St Bartholomew's Hospital where it can still be viewed.

Though he painted and engraved many other subjects it was his moral series which brought him most fame. He was very proud of his Englishness and once signed a painting 'W. Hogarth Anglus Pinxit'.

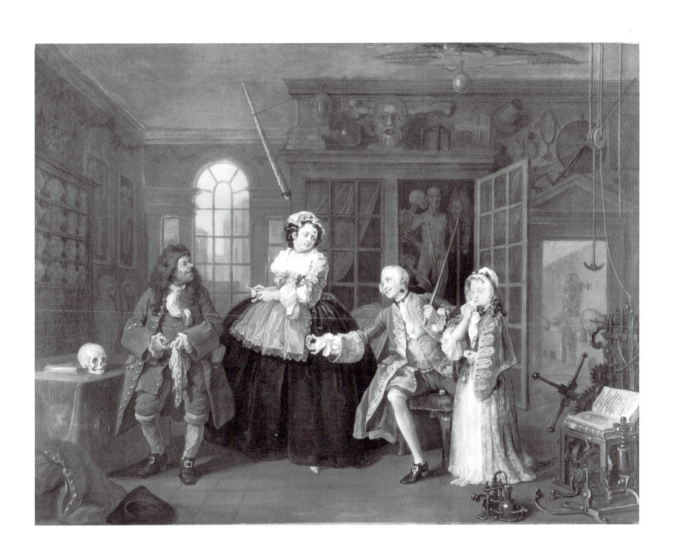

Marriage à la Mode: The Inspection (1743) by William Hogarth (© National Gallery, London).

14

The Apothecary (or The Spice Shop) (1752)
by Pietro Longhi

Pietro Longhi (1702–1785) spent all his life in Venice where he was an acute observer and painter of everyday scenes. There is often a sense of irony in his work but never the biting satire of several contemporary English painters such as Hogarth and Rowlandson. Nevertheless the detail with which he depicted Venetian life in his paintings has provided us with an accurate record of society life in that illustrious city at the moment of its decline. The main characters in his paintings are often engaged in frivolous pursuits under the gaze of their servants who seem to have little sympathy or liking for their employers, though with no strong social or moral judgements.

Here we have the scene of an apothecary's shop where he is examining a young lady, possibly a courtesan. Others are waiting their turn while a young man is heating perhaps a herbal concoction and another is writing out a possible prescription.

The potted plant has been described by some commentators as 'aloes'. However, according to Bentham and Hooker's renowned *British Flora*, the *true* aloes of botanists are in fact liliaceous plants. The term 'aloe' would therefore be incorrect, as this is clearly not a liliaceous plant but an agave plant. This was a recognised symbol of healing at the time and used to ward off plague.

Originally an Apothecary referred in England to anyone who kept a shop of non-perishable commodities including spices and drugs. But in 1617 the Apothecaries were separated from the Grocers and became an independent organisation as the Apothecaries of the City of London. Apothecaries not only sold drugs but also practised medicine. The 1815 Apothecaries Act specified that those who were in effect general practitioners should be trained in medicine and licensed. Those who were not medically trained became restricted to preparing and selling medicines and were referred to as druggists or pharmaceutical chemists. In this painting the Apothecary is clearly involved in both practices: examining the patient as well as recommending and preparing medicine. These dual roles are nicely depicted in the work.

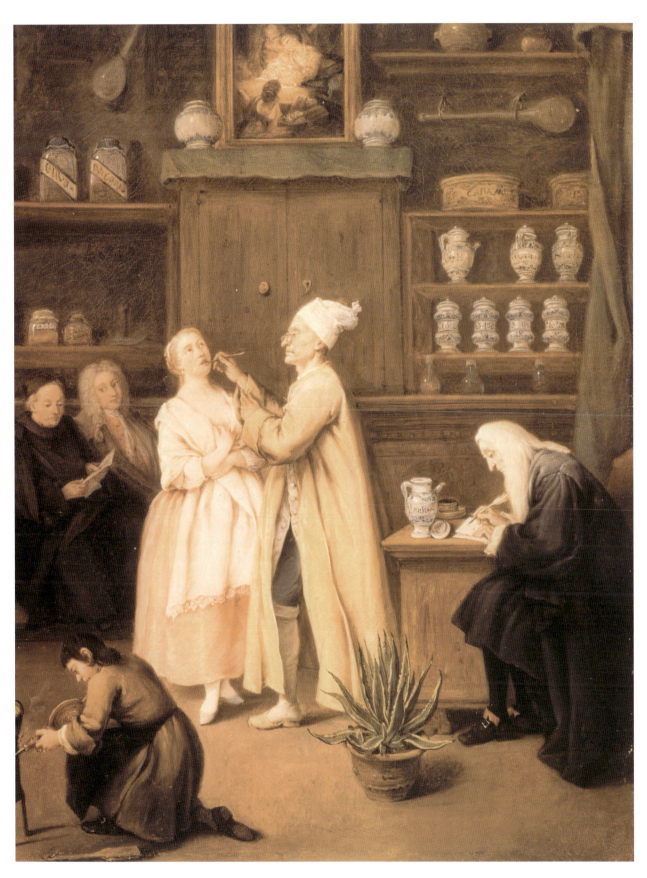

The Apothecary (or *The Spice Shop*) (1752) by Pietro Longhi (Photo Scala, Florence).

15

Dr William Glysson (c 1780–1785)

by Winthrop Chandler

Winthrop Chandler (1747–1790) was descended from a family of early settlers in New England. They were mainly farming stock, successive generations living in and around Woodstock where Chandler Hill is named after them. The artist spent most of his short life amidst the quite solitude of Chandler Hill. From an early age he became interested in painting and at the age of 23 completed an impressive portrait of the Reverend and Mrs Ebenezer Devotion. There is no evidence he took part in the War of Independence though many of his relatives did. Instead he concentrated on his art – mainly portraits and landscape, though with little financial success. He raised a family of five sons and two daughters, but his wife died at an early age in 1789 from tuberculosis, and Chandler himself a year later, possibly from the same disease. He now has a respected place in the annals of early rural American art.

His painting of his brother-in-law, Dr William Glysson (sometimes also referred to as Gleason), is interesting from several points of view. The doctor is clearly successful, being well-dressed with a velvet waistcoat and breeches and wearing spurs, indicating his mode of travel in the country. He also holds a silver-headed cane, the hallmark of a doctor at this time. The heads often contained vinaigrettes or pomanders with supposed disinfectant properties. The artist has taken great care with detail showing exactly how the pulse is taken and where the examining doctor's fingers are placed along the course of the radial artery. The early New England settlers were strongly religious and propriety and modesty were important. This would explain why, in taking the pulse, the patient is shrouded from view within the privacy of a carefully curtained bed. This approach to examining a patient was to persist, at least in many country districts, until the beginning of the nineteenth century.

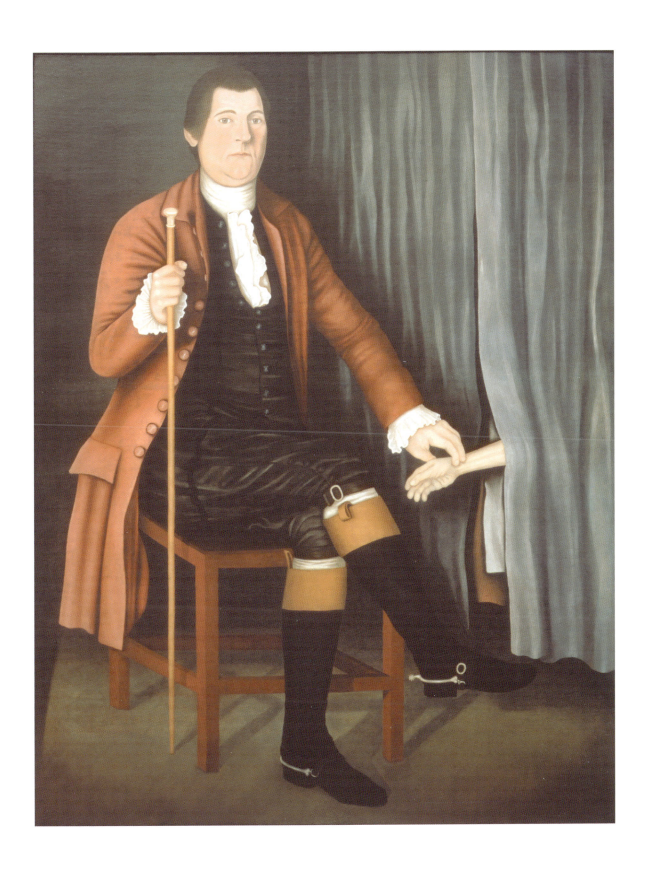

Dr William Glysson (c 1780–1785) by Winthrop Chandler (courtesy of the Ohio Historical Society, Columbus, Ohio).

16

Pinel Frees the Insane from their Chains (1876)

by Tony Robert-Fleury

The care of the mentally ill over the centuries has largely reflected the community's attitude to such illness. Disturbed behaviour was frequently viewed as the result of demonic possession, and the mentally ill were often the subjects of amusement and entertainment (witness Hogarth's 1735 series devoted to The Rake's Progress which depicted patients at the Bethlem Hospital). But by the late eighteenth century these views were changing. For example William Cullen (1710–1790), an Edinburgh physician, believed insanity to be a disease of the nervous system. One of the most influential figures in this regard was Philippe Pinel (1745–1826), a physician and devout Roman Catholic. He had responsibility for the insane at the Bicêtre Hospital in Paris in the early 1790s, at the time of the Revolution. He experimented with reducing mechanical restraints because he believed that the mentally ill needed care and support rather than incarceration. The idea that insanity was the result of disease of the nervous system gradually gained acceptance and later in 1865 in Berlin, Wilhelm Griesinger (1817–1868) became the first Professor of Psychiatry and Neurology, thus emphasising the intellectual importance of this new speciality.

The artist Tony Robert-Fleury (1837–1911) was born and worked all his life in Paris. He became renowned for his large historical compositions, such as this one, and received many awards and honours. Robert-Fleury clearly over-dramatised the event, painted many years later, in which Pinel released some 49 patients from their bondage. Even so this painting has become a well-deserved icon of a very important turning point in the care of the mentally ill.

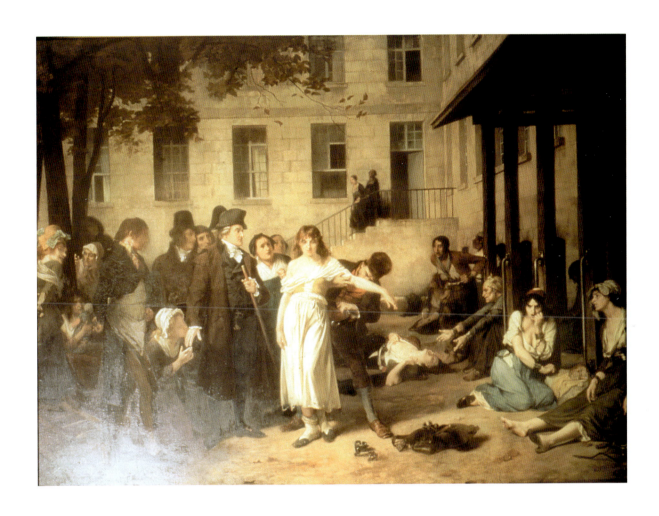

Pinel Frees the Insane from their Chains (1876) by Tony Robert-Fleury (reproduced by kind permission of the Universite Paris V1, Bibliothèque Charcot, Hôpital de la Salpêtrière, Paris).

17

Vaccination (1807)

by Louis-Léopold Boilly

Since earliest times mankind has been afflicted with smallpox, a disease with a high mortality. It spread throughout the world as a result of trade and colonial expansion. For example, in the 16th century it accompanied Cortés in his conquest of Mexico and Pizarro in his conquest of Peru. It was known for some time that the Chinese practice of variolation conferred immunity. This involved the deliberate introduction of a small amount of smallpox matter scratched into the skin or blown up the nose. The technique was praised by many people of eminence including Benjamin Franklin, Voltaire and Catherine the Great. But it was the introduction of vaccination (from the Latin *vacca* for cow) by Edward Jenner (1749–1823) that proved a more agreeable and more effective form of protection.

It had been known for some time that dairy-maids infected with cowpox (a mild infection in humans) became immune to smallpox. This Jenner proved by experimental inoculation of an eight year-old country boy named James Phipps with cowpox material from an infected milkmaid. Then, after an interval of six weeks, he inoculated the boy with smallpox with no effect (such an experiment nowadays would be fraught with ethical problems). He studied several other cases and published the results in his seminal paper, 'An Inquiry into the Causes and Effects of the Variolae Vaccinae' in 1798. At first there were critics (James Gillray depicted vaccinated individuals with cow-like appearances in one of his engravings) and an anti-vaccination campaign was started in England. But the practice soon gained acceptance and spread across the world. Even by 1799 over 5000 individuals in England had been vaccinated, and in France between 1808 and 1811 no less than 1.7 million people were successfully vaccinated. The adoption of the procedure led ultimately to the global eradication of smallpox in 1979, some 200 years after Jenner's publication. Interestingly medical historians have noted that Benjamin Jesty, a Dorset farmer, protected his own family by vaccination some twenty years before Jenner. But he used material directly from an infected cow which at the time raised a great deal of criticism from the Church, whereas Jenner used material from an infected human being, and furthermore made a systematic study of successfully vaccinating more than twenty individuals. Jenner was a physician who had trained under John Hunter and was later elected a Fellow of the Royal Society, not for his work on smallpox however, but for his research on cuckoos.

A number of artists have depicted the act of vaccination: for example Diego Rivera in Mexico, Ernest Board in England, Reinhard Zimmermann in Germany, and several French artists including C.J. Desbordes, Gaston Melingue and here by Louis-Léopold Boilly (1761–1845). Boilly was a popular genre painter whose work was sometimes tinged with a gentle sentimentality. One of his works however was considered to be too erotic and was condemned by the Comité du Salut Public in 1794 at the height of the Terror. Thereafter he reverted to more traditional subjects and was awarded a gold medal at the Paris Salon in 1804 and later admitted to the Légion d'honneur. In this work we see the doctor in his traditional formal attire of the period vaccinating a young child while the other main characters look on, some with concerned interest but others with apprehension. These must well have been the reactions of people at the time.

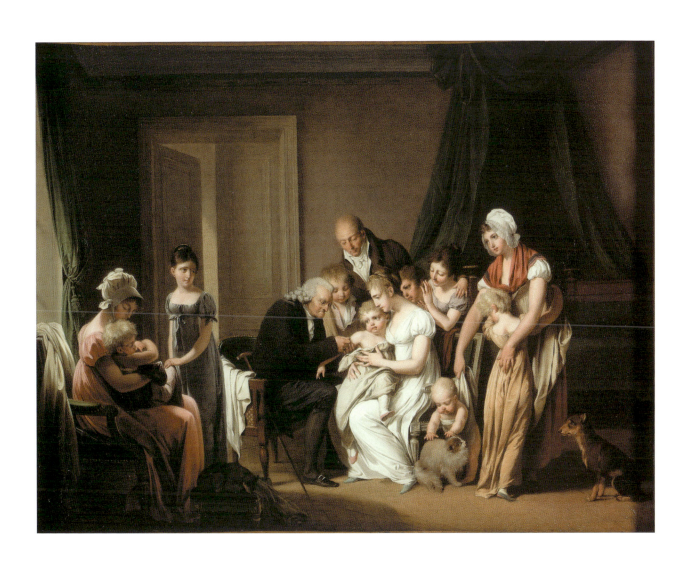

Vaccination (1807) by Louis-Léopold Boilly (The Wellcome Library, London).

18

A Mandarin Doctor Consulting a Patient (19th century)

by Zhou Pei Qun

The history of Chinese medicine can be traced back to writings well over 2000 years ago, with influences over time from India, Tibet and Central and South-East Asia. Traditionally Chinese medicine emphasised a natural and holistic approach to illness. *Yang* and *yin* were conceived as two opposing forces which dominated everything in the world from astronomical phenomena to health and disease. Though *yang* and *yin* were opposites, they were not seen as in conflict but complementary. Around such ideas the Chinese developed a complex, essentially philosophical and supernatural approach to the causes of disease. Natural remedies, massage and acupuncture were important elements in treatment.

Pulse-taking was an essential aspect of assessing a patient, as we see in this 19th century illustration. It was elaborated into a complex art with palpation of the radial pulse carried out at different depths and locations. The physician also considered and carefully noted the patient's complexion, breathing, emotional state, fever and so on. But the scope for examining the patient was severely restricted because of modesty which prevented exposing the female body. In fact miniature statuettes modelled in ivory, porcelain or wood were used by women to indicate to the physician the site on her body which caused pain or discomfort. Physicians were unable to relate their detailed observations to lesions of internal organs until later in the 19th century. Nevertheless an important legacy of traditional Chinese medicine is seen with today's emphasis on an holistic approach to the patient.

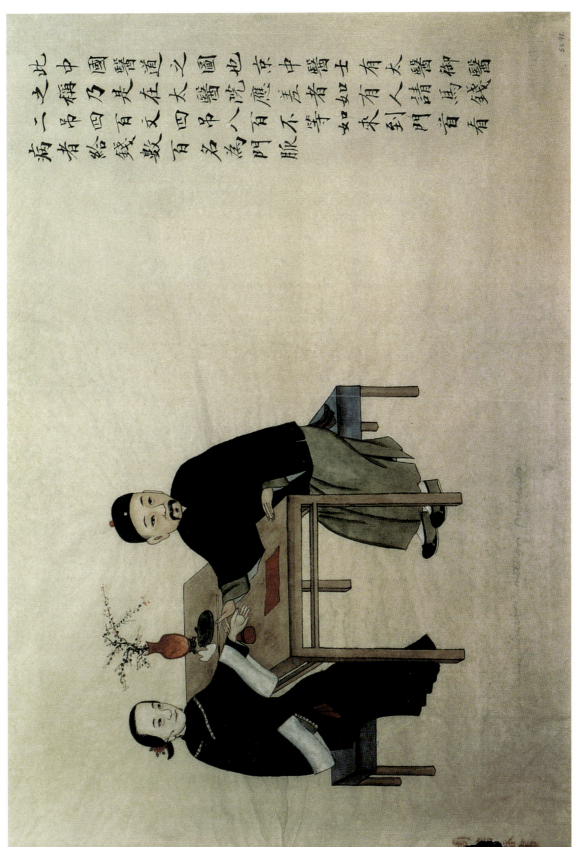

醫錢春有醫

御醫有大醫御醫

請人詣門看

未到門

有大醫

士有

中應差者

醫者如以

中醫士

道之應人院門為

圖書名

之四書文數百

國四百錢數百

中書乃圓

此二病者給

A Mandarin Doctor Consulting a Patient (19th century) by Zhou Pei Qun (The Wellcome Library, London).

19

George Washington in His Last Illness, Attended by Doctors Craik and Brown

(c 1800) Coloured Engraving

George Washington (1732–1799) was elected first President of the United States of America under the new Constitution in 1789, and as such much has been written about his life, including his medical history. He was born in Bridges Creek, Westmoreland County in Virginia, of English immigrant stock. He was a healthy, hard-working lad renowned for his honesty, though the story of his admitting to cutting down his father's cherry tree probably had little basis in fact. He became an officer in the militia and later the colonial army. In 1759 he married a rich young widow, Martha Custis. After the War of Independence he became President for two terms, but refused a further term and returned to his estate in Mount Vernon, where he died on 14 December 1799. Henry Lee's words at the time of his death remain his finest epitaph: 'First in war, first in peace, first in the hearts of his fellow citizens.'

He suffered much from tooth problems probably as a result of pyorrhoea and dental caries and throughout the War of Independence he had constant toothache. By 1796 he had lost his last tooth – a lower premolar. The difficulty of wearing various ill-fitting contraptions to replace his missing teeth was a constant problem and made clear speech difficult. It was however his last illness which has attracted much attention by medical historians. In this picture we see his attentive doctors in typical colonial dress of the time taking the dying patient's pulse with his grieving wife in the background. This was at a time when blood-letting or phlebotomy was widely practised for all manner of illnesses. Washington himself suffered from what may have been a streptococcal infection following a winter's ride on his farm in Virginia. He instructed his doctors to bleed him copiously, which they did. Elish Dick, the youngest of the three doctors who attended the President had cautioned against massive bleeding but he was over-ruled by the two older physicians. The President's death followed two days later and significantly added to the growing discontent with the procedure which was thereafter gradually abandoned by the profession.

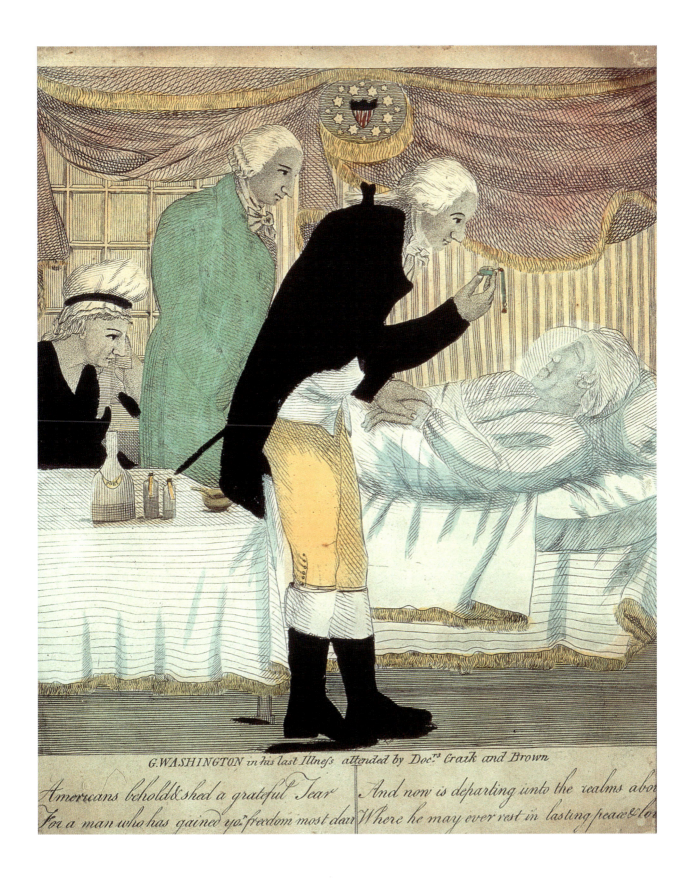

G.WASHINGTON *in his last Illness* attended by Doc.ʳˢ *Craik and Brown*

Americans behold & shed a grateful Tear   And now is departing unto the realms abo
For a man who has gained yoᵘ freedom most dar   Where he may ever rest in lasting peace & lo

George Washington in His Last Illness, Attended by Doctors Craik and Brown (c 1800). (Olds Collection #96, negative no. 46066. Collection of the New-York Historical Society).

20

The Consultation or Last Hope (1808)

by Thomas Rowlandson

The medical profession, at least in Britain, was not regarded particularly well in the eighteenth and early nineteenth centuries. It was ridiculed and lampooned in art by Hogarth and subsequently by others including James Gillray, George Cruikshank and particularly Thomas Rowlandson (1756–1827). The latter's etchings and water-colours were especially critical of the profession, quackery and the innocent gullibility of patients.

Rowlandson was born in London and at the age of 16 went to Paris to study for two years. When he returned to England he began to paint serious subjects. But he was an inveterate gambler and after squandering all the money he inherited from a French aunt, he turned to producing a flood of material largely concerned with everyday life, at least a hundred with medical themes. He had many medical friends and a frequent supper companion was a Dr John Wolcot who probably provided him with many first-hand ideas for drawings.

The late Roy Porter, the medical historian, has argued that medical practitioners at the time were often viewed by the populace as being no more than players in the social scene. Their diagnostic capabilities were limited and there were no treatments apart from emetics, purgatives, leeching and blood-letting. Furthermore careful physical examination of patients did not become standard practice until at least the mid-19th century.

In this painting of Rowlandson's there are no less than five practitioners surrounding the patient, apparently engaged in consultation while others await their turn. On the mantelpiece are many tried and unsuccessful remedies and the nurse is fast asleep. In the face of severe life-threatening illness there was little the physician could do except take the patient's pulse, pontificate and contemplate his fee. All this is mercilessly depicted in Rowlandson's work.

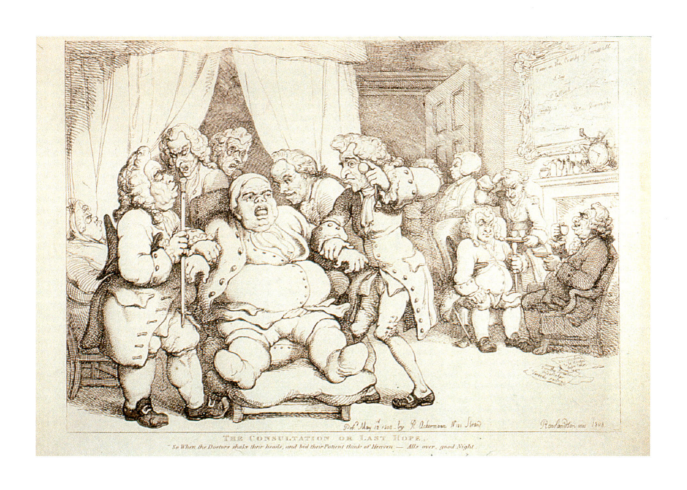

The Consultation or Last Hope (1808) by Thomas Rowlandson.

21

Laënnec Listening to the Chest of a Patient (c 1910)

by Ernest Board

The second half of the nineteenth century was the real beginning of medical science, with the invention of many important diagnostic tools. These included the ophthalmoscope by Charles Babbage in 1847, later improved by Hermann von Helmholtz; the laryngoscope by Manuel Garcia in 1854–5; and the clinical thermometer by Thomas Allbutt around 1870. But the simplest and one of the most important innovations was Rene Laënnec's (1781–1826) introduction of the stethoscope in 1816. At first this was no more than a rolled-up piece of stiff paper, and later a simple wooden cylinder. This monaural device was subsequently replaced by the present-day binaural stethoscope, introduced by the American, George P. Cammann, in 1852. Laënnec's instrument allowed him to diagnose many pulmonary diseases, such as bronchitis, pneumonia and above all pulmonary tuberculosis. Ironically, he himself died of pulmonary tuberculosis in 1826 at the early age of 45, just a few years after the publication of his celebrated work, *Traité de l'Auscultation Médiate.*

A number of painters have attempted over the years to catch the importance of Laënnec's invention in art. Théobold Chartran painted the subject in the 1880s, some years after Laënnec's death, showing him at a patient's bedside at the Necker Hospital in Paris. And in 1945 Robert Thom, an American painter and illustrator born in Grand Rapids, Michigan, also painted the subject. The illustration here is by the English painter Ernest Board (1877–1934). He was born in Worcester and studied at the Royal College of Art and the Royal Academy Schools. He exhibited at the Royal Academy on many occasions and made a special study of historical events and portraits of well-known historical figures, including John and Sebastian Cabot the explorers, Rhazes the Arabian physician, Dr Edward Jenner performing his first vaccination, and this one of Laënnec using a simple monaural cylinder to enhance the sounds of the patient's breathing. The artist has captured the intense expression of the physician as he attempts to interpret the sounds he hears as a reflection of the underlying lung pathology in a patient who is thin and pale and probably suffering from pulmonary tuberculosis.

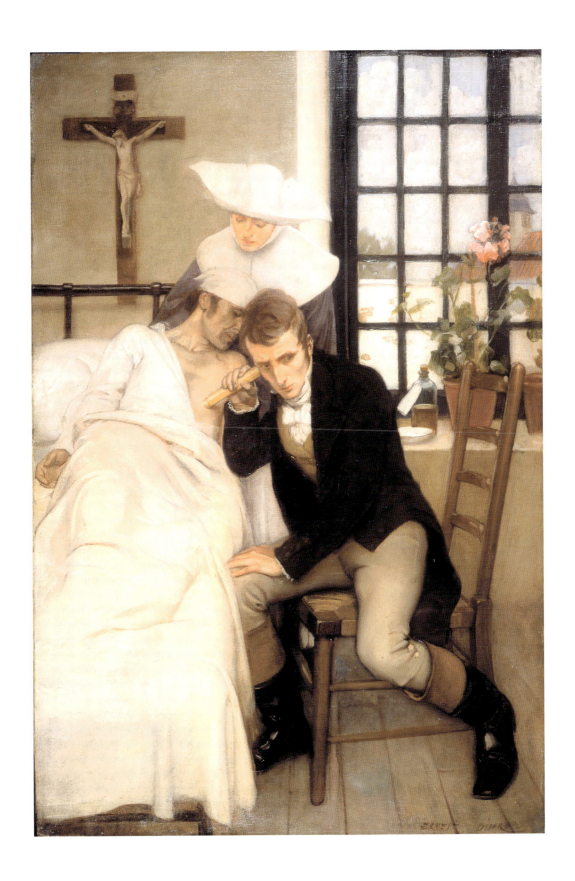

Laënnec Listening to the Chest of a Patient (c 1910) by Ernest Board (private collection, UK).

22

Self-portrait with Dr Arrieta (1820)

by Francisco de Goya

Goya was the greatest painter of 18th century Spain and undoubtedly among the most famous artists of all time. Francisco José de Goya y Lucientes was born on 30 March 1746 in the small village of Fuendetodos, near Saragossa, where he later became an apprentice to José Luzan, at that time the leading artist of Saragossa. There he also met the painter Francisco Bayeu whose sister he later married. Bayeu's success eventually led him to the Royal Court in Madrid where Goya subsequently joined him. But it was not until Goya was in his mid-30s that he began to gain recognition as a renowned artist, and in 1780 was elected a member of the Madrid Academy. In 1789 Charles IV was crowned and Goya became one of the royal painters and later, Principal Painter to the King, a promotion which he marked by adding the aristocratic 'de' to his name.

However at the age of 47 in 1792 he developed a serious illness, the nature of which is still controversial. According to contemporary accounts, he suffered temporary loss of balance, the right side of his body was paralysed and he was unable to walk, and he developed a temporary partial blindness. This was clearly an acute neurological disorder and it now seems likely it could have been the result of a viral infection, perhaps even Vogt-Koyanagi-Harada syndrome. He retired to Cadiz for several months until he recovered though he remained permanently deaf. This harrowing illness left an indelible mark on his later paintings which often include macabre subjects. In fact some art historians have argued that this marked a change in art in general away from its public and social function toward pictorial revelations of an artist's subjective feelings. But Goya also continued to paint many conventional subjects including a number of renowned portraits such as that of the Duke of Wellington in 1812.

A serious illness struck him again in 1819 at the age of 73 but he recovered under the care of the Madrid physician, Dr Eugenio Garcia Arrieta. The latter's caring attention and Goya's prostration are vividly depicted in this double portrait which the artist painted in gratitude to his doctor for his recovery. The dark figures depicted in the background perhaps represent harbingers of death.

After recovery, his artistic ability and enthusiasm returned and remained undiminished until on the 16th of April 1828 he suffered a paralytic stroke and died aged 82.

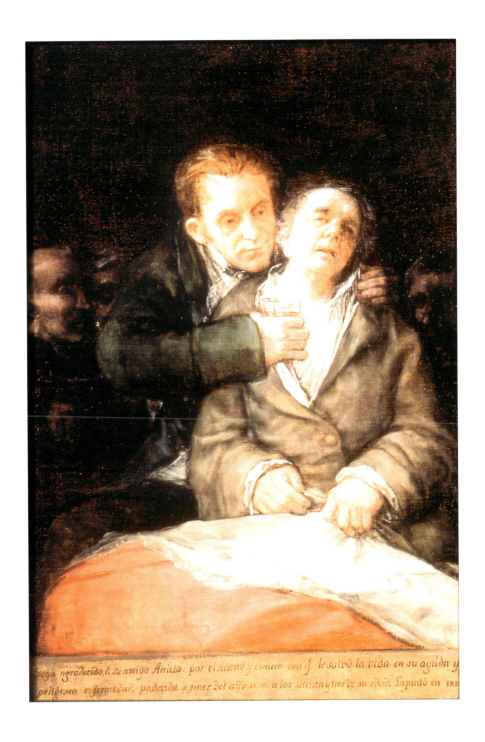

Self-portrait with Dr Arrieta (1820) by Francisco de Goya (reproduced by kind permission of The Minneapolis Institute of Arts. The Ethel Morrison van Derlip Fund).

23

The Doctor Robert Macaire (1836)

by Honoré Daumier

In the 19th century there were many famous physicians practising in Paris. These included Laënnec, the inventor of the stethoscope, Récamier, who first recognised the process of metastasis, Duchenne and Charcot, pioneers in neurology, and of course the new generation of experimental physiologists, notably Magendie and Claude Bernard. But as in all medical societies there were also the charlatans, the avaricious and the boastful, and it is they whom Honoré Daumier (1808–1879) satirised in many of his lithographs and drawings.

This particular work features a patient consulting a Dr Robert Macaire. The latter was named after a fictional character of ridicule in a play current in Paris at the time. Daumier often used this character as a symbol in his attacks not only on doctors but also dentists, surgeons, unscrupulous lawyers and bankers. In his lampooning of doctors he could be just as critical of the patient, particularly the imaginary invalid. The subtitle of this particular work reads '*For heaven's sake, don't take this sickness lightly! … Believe me, drink water, lots of water … rub the bones of your legs … and come to see me often … that won't impoverish you … my consultations are free … Now, you owe me 20 francs for these two bottles …. (this includes 10 centimes deposit on each container).*'

In 1832 Daumier's representation of King Louis Philippe as Gargantua landed him in prison. And though his works were admired by famous artists of the time, including Delacroix, Millet and Corot, he remained poor throughout his life. He became blind through cataracts in old age and it was the failure of surgical treatment which caused Monet considerable concern when years later he also faced the same problem. In Monet's case however surgery subsequently proved successful.

Daumier seems otherwise to have had remarkably good health until the winter of 1878 when he suffered a stroke from which he never recovered. He died shortly afterwards in 1879.

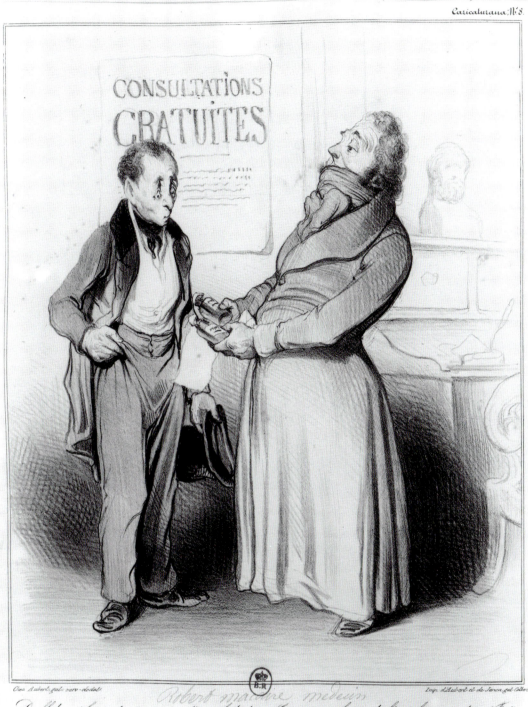

The Doctor Robert Macaire (1836) by Honoré Daumier (reproduced by kind permission of the Bibliothèque nationale de France).

24

A Medicine Man Curing a Patient (c 1850)
by C. Schuessele after a work by Captain S. Eastman

Shamans, witch doctors or medicine-men foster the belief that sickness is related to supernatural events or evil spirits. In certain cave paintings in France some 17,000 years ago, men are depicted wearing animal head-dresses and performing ritualistic dances which may well represent the earliest record of Shamans. The practice still continues today in some North American Indian and North Asian tribes and aspects of these supernatural beliefs persist in certain other communities, even in the West.

The role of the Shaman combines those of healer, sorcerer, soothsayer, educator and priest. Usually a man, he is believed to possess powers to heal the sick, ensure fertility or a good harvest or a successful hunt. His rituals involve dances, fetishes, amulets to protect against black magic, and talismans for good luck. He may draw on certain objects (shells, bones, entrails) or rely on the evocation of a trance to determine the cause of an illness. The beliefs are often deeply held and the effects on the sick person may well be the result of heightened suggestibility and even be psychotherapeutic in some cases.

This illustration is a chromolithograph by Christian Schuessele (1824–1879), a French-born artist who emigrated to Philadelphia in 1848, after a work by Captain Seth Eastman (1808–1875). Eastman attended the US Military Academy at West Point and subsequently was stationed at various military forts in North America. Here he came into intimate contact with North American Indians, carefully recording their everyday activities and he illustrated a major text on the subject (H.R. Schoolcraft's *Information Respecting the History, Condition and Prospects of the Indian Tribes of the United States*, Philadelphia, 1851–1857). He had little formal training but he nevertheless provided an invaluable record of the life of the American Indian at the time. In this illustration, the medicine man has been summoned to the patient's tepee and sits shaking a rattle made from a dried gourd containing beads or stones, presumably to charm the evil spirits believed to be causing the illness of the patient lying on the bed in the background.

According to Mary Eastman, Captain Eastman's wife, in her book concerned with the life and legends of the Sioux Indians published in 1840, the medicine man would then proceed either to draw out the evil spirit with his mouth or if he thought some animal, fowl or fish possessed the sick person, an effigy was made of bark and then young men of the tribe instructed to shoot it with arrows and the remains collected and burned. At this point the ceremony ceased and the hope was the patient would recover.

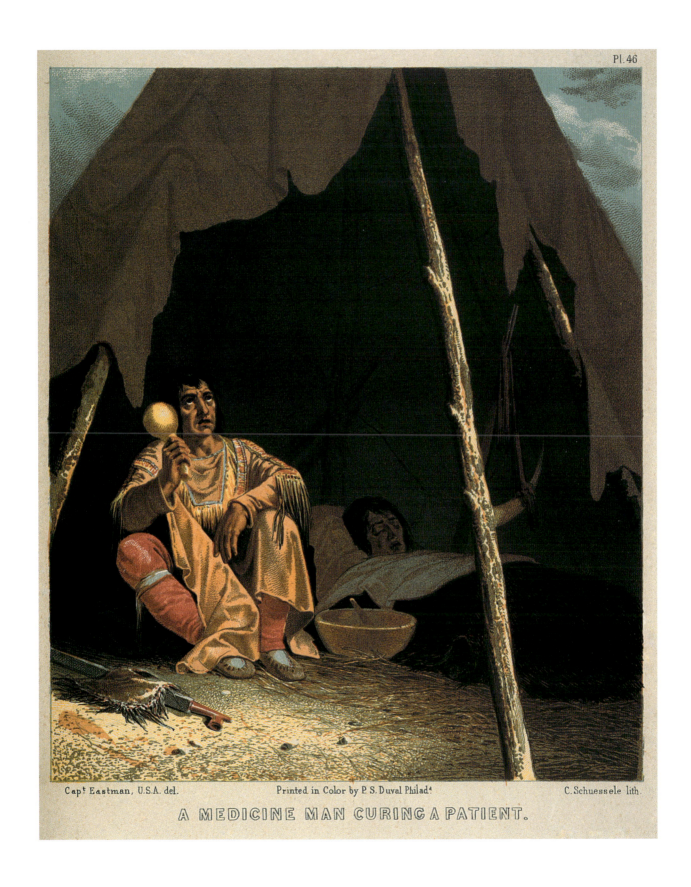

Pl. 46

Cap.ᵗ Eastman, U.S.A. del.   Printed in Color by P.S.Duval Philad.ᵃ   C.Schuessele lith.

A MEDICINE MAN CURING A PATIENT.

A Medicine Man Curing a Patient (c 1850) Chromolithograph by C. Schuessele after a work by Captain S. Eastman (The Wellcome Library, London).

25

The Mission of Mercy: Florence Nightingale Receiving the Wounded at Scutari (1857)

by Jerry Barrett

Jerry Barrett (1824–1906) was a Victorian historical and genre painter who exhibited at the Royal Academy many times between 1851 and 1883. The meticulous detail and his depiction of scenes associated with heightened patriotic feelings around the time of the Crimean War (1854–6) made Barrett's work very popular.

This and an earlier painting (*Victoria and Albert Visiting the Crimean Wounded at Chatham Hospital*) were based on sketches made in Scutari and on portraits made in London. This painting is especially interesting because of the emphasis on Florence Nightingale (1820–1910) whose experiences of the atrocious conditions in British hospitals during the Crimean War led her not only to offer aid and comfort to the wounded but to reorganise the entire nursing care of the sick. When she and her assistants arrived in November 1854 there were nearly 2000 wounded lying in filthy rat-infested wards and the mortality rate was around 50 percent. But after her reorganisation and insistence on absolute cleanliness in the care of the wounded the mortality had fallen to just over 1 percent. Thereafter she dedicated her life to hospital care in general and the role of training nurses. Her own 'School for Nurses' was opened at St Thomas' Hospital in London in 1860. Her system for training nurses gradually spread throughout the world: to Sweden and Australia in 1867, to the United States in 1873, to Canada in 1874 and Denmark in 1897.

In this painting immediately to the right of Florence Nightingale, the central figure, stand Selina and Charles Bracebridge, who were her old friends and assisted her in Scutari. To the left is the Reverend Mother Mary Clare, by the inner door another nurse (Miss Tebbut), and kneeling by the stretcher case a Mrs Roberts, one of Nightingale's most loyal nurses. Several others are also identifiable in this work including the painter himself looking down on the scene from the window. Florence Nightingale based her pioneering work in health care reform on statistics which she considered essential. At the time Francis Galton, a renowned biometrician and early human geneticist, was recognised as an authority in social statistics. For a time the two corresponded. Her hope was to recruit his support for an endowed professorship in the subject at Oxford. Unfortunately sufficient funds were not forthcoming and the idea floundered. In any event her international renown was firmly established as a reforming pioneer in the training of professional nurses for the care of the sick.

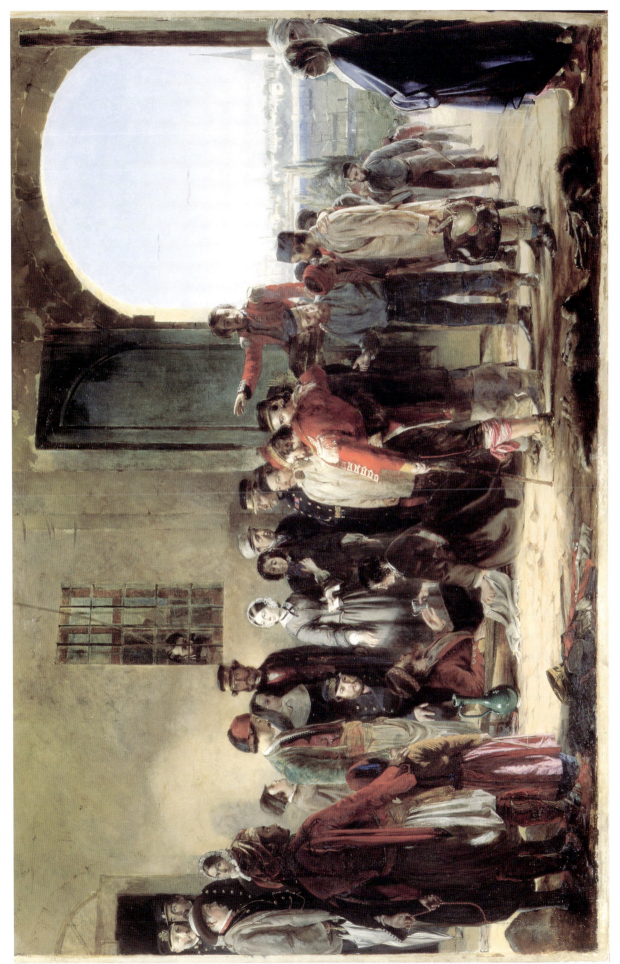

The Mission of Mercy: Florence Nightingale Receiving the Wounded at Scutari (1857) by Jerry Barrett (by courtesy of the National Portrait Gallery, London).

26

The Foundling Restored to its Mother (1858)

by Emma Brownlow

The unwanted child was a major problem in society up until relatively recently when effective contraception became available, adoption agencies were established and, perhaps most significantly, single mothers became socially more acceptable. In the past the social stigma of an illegitimate child could force a mother to abandon her infant. In Victorian London the streets swarmed with unwanted children, often reduced to begging and stealing or occupied in menial jobs and sleeping rough in doors and alleyways. Such children could also become the wards of unscrupulous establishments. Charles Dickens often refers to such children and describes and ridicules these establishments in his novels. The public conscience was deeply disturbed, which led to attempts to rectify the situation with the founding of various charitable organisations such as Dr Barnado's Homes and the Thomas Coram Hospital. The latter was supported by a number of artists and musicians, including Handel.

Emma Brownlow (or Mrs Emma Brownlow King) was born in 1832 and died in 1905. She was the daughter of John Brownlow who had himself been a foundling in the Coram Hospital in 1800 and had risen to become the Secretary to the Governors. Emma Brownlow grew up in the Hospital and was an eyewitness to the way the children were cared for. In this painting we are in the Secretary's office with John Brownlow supervising a foundling child being reunited with her mother. The mother's original receipt lies on the floor along with a box of toys. On the left the foundling, now a little girl, is being led by an older girl, also an orphan, and both are wearing the Hospital's uniform. On the wall behind the Secretary are several pictures including March to Finchley by Hogarth, himself a benefactor and later Governor of the Hospital. For those children lucky enough to get into the Hospital, life seems to have been a very happy one based on Christian virtues, in stark contrast to that of the street children outside.

The painter herself had no formal training but began drawing at an early age and later regularly exhibited her paintings at the Royal Academy. She painted various domestic scenes as well as many based on her travels in Europe. But it was her paintings of life at the Hospital for which she is perhaps best remembered nowadays.

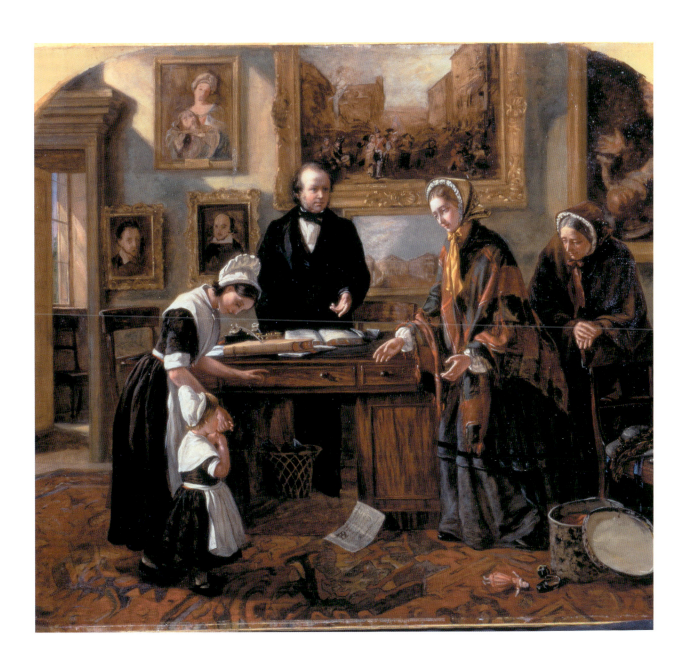

The Foundling Restored to its Mother (1858) by Emma Brownlow (Coram Foundling Museum, London).

28

The Student (c 1860s)

by Francisco Oller y Cestero

There have been very few paintings of doctors in training. One by the Russian painter Leonid Pasternak (1862–1945) in the Musée d'Orsay shows a group of students studying before an examination. In this painting by Oller y Cestero, also in the Musée d'Orsay, the artist has captured the domestic atmosphere of a medical student studying at home in Paris. It has been suggested that the man was a Cuban medical student and painter, Aguiar. His companion is engrossed in sewing, perhaps implying she is supporting him through his studies – a not uncommon practice even nowadays. The student is reading a textbook, probably anatomy since he is holding a skull in his right hand. There is a large and conspicuous coffee pot on his table suggesting the need to concentrate and stay awake.

This is also an interesting painting from an artistic point of view, for Oller was influenced by both the French Realists, such as Gustav Courbet, as well as the emerging Impressionists Camille Pissarro and Paul Cézanne. He was born (1833) and died (1917) in Puerto Rico. This was formerly a Spanish colony and he first studied art in Madrid. But in 1858 he went to Paris for further training and this led to the bright airiness of his work so characteristic of the Impressionists. After a stay in Puerto Rico from 1865 to 1873, he returned again to Paris for a decade, but settled permanently in Puerto Rico in 1884. He became renowned for paintings of his country and sought to create specifically Puerto Rican art associated with the country's rising nationalism. Interestingly this painting was later bought by Dr Paul Gachet, an early patron of the Impressionists and a homeopathic practitioner with a particular interest in mental health, who later cared for van Gogh. Van Gogh in turn painted two memorable portraits of the doctor himself, one now in a private collection in Japan, the other in the Musée d'Orsay, Paris.

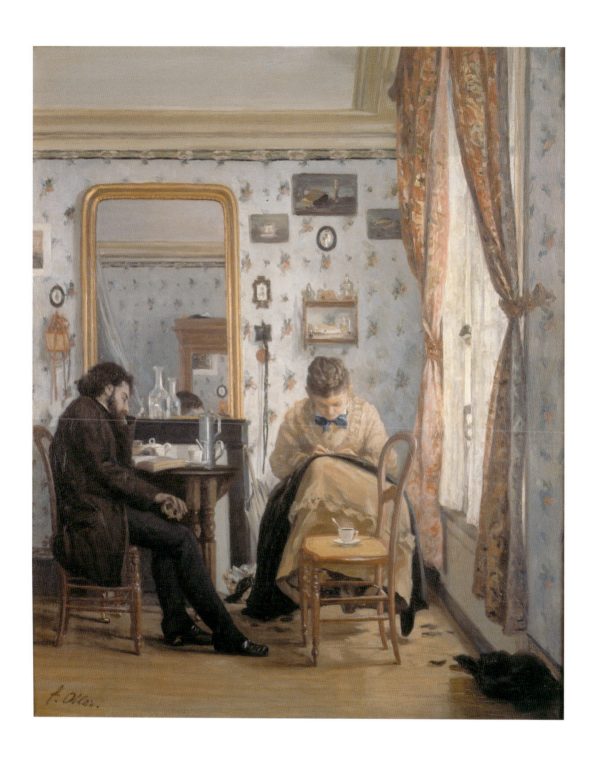

The Student (c 1860s) by Francisco Oller y Cestero (© Photo RMN – Hervé Lewandowski).

29

Doubtful Hope (1875)

by Frank Holl

There was much poverty and sickness in Victorian England. One artist who made a particular study of this was Frank Holl, who was born in London in 1845 and died at the early age of 43, purportedly from overwork. He came from a family of engravers and at 15 he entered the Royal Academy Schools where he won a silver medal in 1862 and a gold medal in 1863. With a travelling scholarship he toured widely in Europe and was particularly impressed with Holland, a love which he later shared with his wife. Here he became especially interested in the work of the Dutch painter, Jozef Israels, who often painted poverty-stricken peasantry as did Van Gogh in his early work (e.g. *The Potato Eaters*). Van Gogh expressly admired Holl's work *Deserted – A Foundling*.

Up until 1879 when Holl turned more to portrait painting, his main themes were everyday poverty in Britain, maternal grief and infant death. This sad, sombre character of his work has been attributed to his being a lonely, delicate and often ailing child brought up in a narrow and frugal household. Whatever the explanation, these early paintings are depressingly moving. In this painting a poor young mother sits forlornly holding her baby wrapped in rags and waits for the chemist to prepare a medicine which from her expression, and also reflected in the title of the work, is unlikely to have any benefit. An assistant routinely writes out the bill. Holl took great care with authenticity and an actual chemist's shop in Camden Town provided the background to the painting with its wooden fittings and rows of jars and bottles. This was a time when the infant mortality rate per 1000 live births was around 150 compared with a figure of less than 10 nowadays. The artist has succeeded completely in capturing the atmosphere and the grief of the mother at a time when such events were not uncommon.

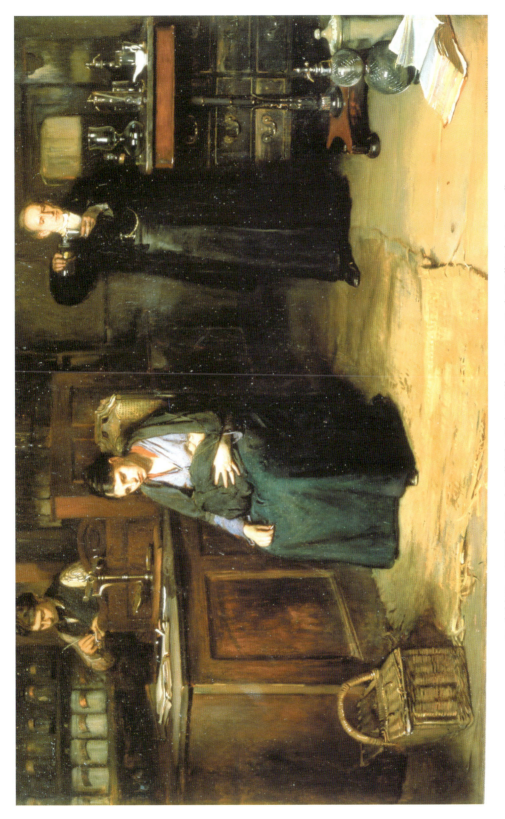

Doubtful Hope (1875) by Frank Holl (The Forbes Collection, New York © All Rights Reserved).

30

A Visit to Aesculapius (1880)

by Sir Edward Poynter

The ancient Greeks associated healing powers with their legendary god Asclepius (or Asklepios), later adopted by the Romans as Aesculapius. It could be that Asclepius may originally have been based on a real person who attended the sick, but essentially he was a mythological character. Even to the present day his serpent-entwined staff is often used as an emblem for the caring professions and organisations. In this painting by Sir Edward Poynter (1836–1919) the scene is based on a poem by Elizabeth Thomas Watson. Aesculapius is being consulted by Venus, identified by the doves which are her attributes, who has a thorn in her foot. She is accompanied by the Three Graces.

Poynter was born in Paris of Huguenot ancestry. He studied in Rome and later Paris and London. In 1871 he became Slade Professor of Fine Art at University College London and subsequently director of the National Gallery and from 1896 to 1918 president of the Royal Academy. He was a fine draughtsman and his paintings, often of biblical and classical themes, were much valued in their day.

Of course any impression of Aesculapius has to be purely imaginative. But in this painting Poynter was more concerned with depicting the female figure. Victorian prudery however frowned on such work. So British artists of the time who wanted to paint the female nude had to resort to various devices in order to avoid public censure. These devices included the use of classical themes with nudes being painted in pale alabaster-like colours in order to resemble statues, flesh colours being avoided. Furthermore the nudes themselves had to have their gaze turned away from the observer to prevent any possibility of the latter becoming intimidated! All these devices are beautifully illustrated in Poynter's painting.

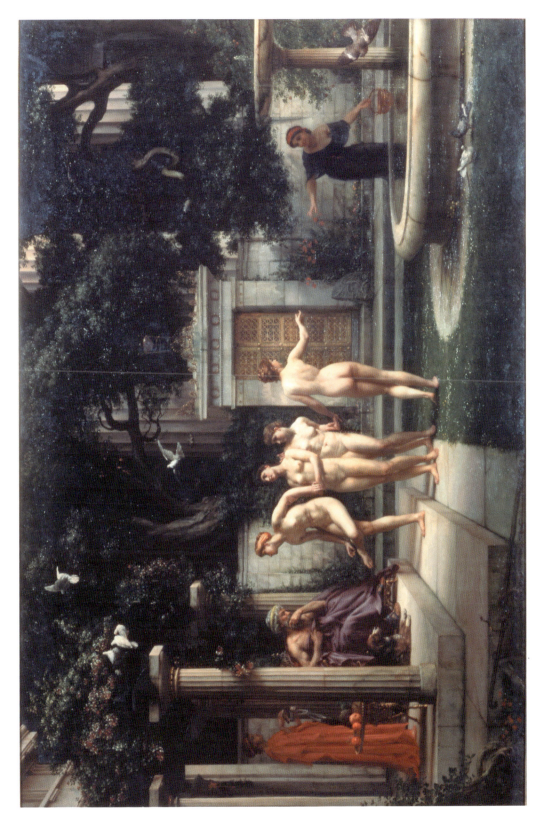

31

Clinical Lesson at the Salpêtrière (c 1887)

by Pierre-André Brouillet

Jean-Martin Charcot (1825–1893) was essentially a clinician with a particular interest in diseases of the nervous system. He shunned animal experiments and his contributions to the subject were exclusively from detailed and careful study of patients mainly at the Salpêtrière Hospital – a large public hospital in Paris. His many and important contributions to neurology included describing the clinical manifestations of multiple sclerosis, and delineating amyotrophic lateral sclerosis. Various other conditions with which his name is still associated include Charcot-Marie-Tooth disease, Charcot's joint and Charcot's triad. But quite apart from these conditions he was also renowned for his clinical presentations which attracted much attention from the profession at the time.

It was in such an atmosphere that he demonstrated hysterical behaviour in patients and the effects of hypnosis. In this illustration of one of Charcot's Friday lectures we see such a dramatic demonstration. Later it came to be acknowledged that both hysteria and hypnosis were not neurological conditions but the results of heightened suggestibility. The rapt attention of his audience has been captured by the artist, Pierre-André Brouillet (1857–c 1914/1920). Not a great deal is known about him other than that he painted portraits, scenes of everyday life and various historical events, some with a medical theme as here. However he must have taken much care with his work as several of Charcot's contemporaries at the Salpêtrière can be identified in the painting though not all of whom were physicians. The physicians include, for example, Babinski (supporting the patient), Gilles de la Tourette (seated in the middle wearing an apron), Pierre Marie (seated third from the right) and Charcot's son (leaning against the window with his arms folded) who was a 20-year-old medical student at the time and later became an internationally renowned explorer. Freud had a copy of this work in his study in Vienna and brought it with him when he fled to England in 1938. Incidentally Charcot himself was an accomplished artist and often produced detailed sketches of his patients.

Case presentations have now become a well-established means of medical teaching both to students and to post-graduates as in this illustration.

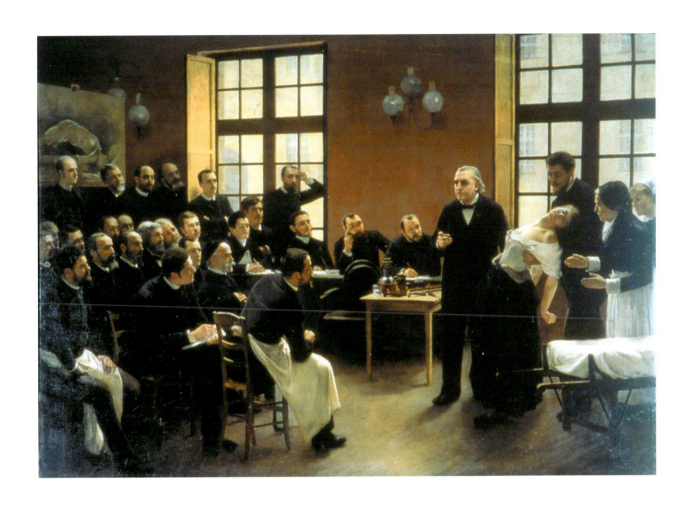

Clinical Lesson at the Salpêtrière (c 1887) by Pierre-André Brouillet (reproduced by kind permission of the Musée d'Histoire de la Médicine, Paris).

32

The Hospital at Arles (1889)

by Vincent van Gogh

The details of the life of Vincent van Gogh (1853–1890) have been well documented and have become almost a legend. He was the son of a Dutch pastor and grew up in a strict Calvinistic background. After a brief period employed by picture dealers in the Hague, London and Paris, then teaching in England and working in a bookshop in Holland, he began studying for the Church. He became a missionary in a coal-mining district in Belgium where he lived in great poverty with his parishioners. But eventually he left the Church in 1880 and took up painting, being largely self-taught. In 1888 he left for Arles in the South of France. This proved to be the most productive period of his life but unfortunately it was also the time that his behaviour became erratic culminating in periodic attacks of insanity and ultimately in 1890 in his committing suicide. The cause of his mental breakdown has been the subject of much speculation which includes lead poisoning from his paints, temporal lobe epilepsy, and the effects of alcohol and prolonged exposure to strong sunlight outdoors. But the most likely explanation now seems to be that he suffered from a serious depressive disorder.

During his periodic attacks of mental illness he was cared for in the asylums in Arles and at Saint-Rémy, the former being the subject of this work which he painted while he was a patient. In letters to his brother Theo at the time, he reveals that he felt a prisoner in a world of strange people and refers to this painting as ' ... a study of the mad [sic] ward at the Arles Hospital.' It is hard to imagine that this was painted in a region of France renowned for its bright sunlight. The interior of the ward is dark and forbidding. There is little apparent communication between the figures in the foreground. They all seem lost in their own thoughts as they gather around the stove. The isolation and loneliness of each individual patient must also have been emphasised by their apparent separation in curtained cubicles. The crucifix on the far wall is central to the theme of the hospital in which the care of the sick is under the aegis of the Church and carried out by nursing sisters.

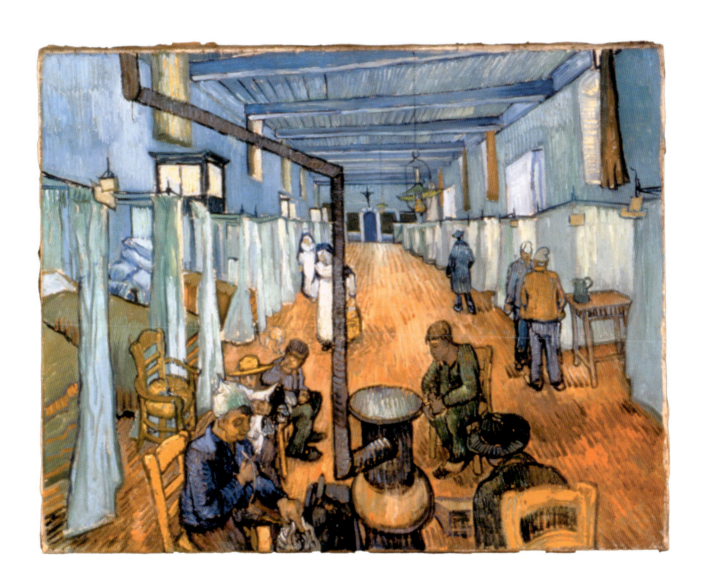

The Hospital at Arles (1889) by Vincent van Gogh (reproduced by kind permission of the Oskar Reinhart Collection, 'Am Römerholz', Winterthur, Switzerland).

33

The Doctor (c 1891)

by Sir Luke Fildes

This is perhaps one of the most famous and most reproduced medical paintings of all time. In the US alone more than a million prints were made and it was reproduced in a postage stamp in 1947. It was commissioned by the wealthy English sugar merchant Sir Henry Tate as one of the original 57 pictures in the Gallery he founded in 1891 where it still hangs. Apparently Tate had merely requested an English subject but the painter immediately decided on *The Doctor*. Despite the popularity in Victorian England of his paintings Fildes never became one of the Great English Painters. In fact many standard works on the history of the subject only make passing reference to him.

Early in his career Samuel Luke Fildes (1843–1927) belonged to a group of late Victorian painters who could be considered social realists. They frequently portrayed scenes of working class life, factories and workhouses. At this time Fildes' painting of the homeless queuing for overnight accommodation, *Applicants for Admission to a Casual Ward* (1874), created a sensation at the Royal Academy. His interest in such subjects had been shaped by his grandmother who had adopted and raised him from childhood and who herself had been wounded at the Peterloo Massacre. However apart from *The Doctor* none of his later attempts at social realism made much impact and he turned to the much more lucrative theme of portrait painting.

His painting *The Doctor* was very carefully and meticulously constructed. The artist spent a week in Devon sketching fishermen's cottages in preparation for the picture. From these sketches he constructed a full-sized replica of a cottage interior in his studio. The painting was clearly a response to the loss of his own little son, Phillip, on Christmas morning some years previously. At the time doctors could do little for their young patients with infectious diseases such as diphtheria, scarlet fever and meningitis. They could only watch and try to console the parents (here father stands by his wife who cradles her head in her hands). This has been a long night, the dawn light is filtering through the cottage window, a half-empty bottle of medicine stands on the table, the child sleeps and all wait. A poignant scene reproduced by Fildes with obvious feeling and a graphic reminder of the practice and impotence of medicine before the era of polypharmacy and technological innovations. But the image of the caring, vigilant doctor remains.

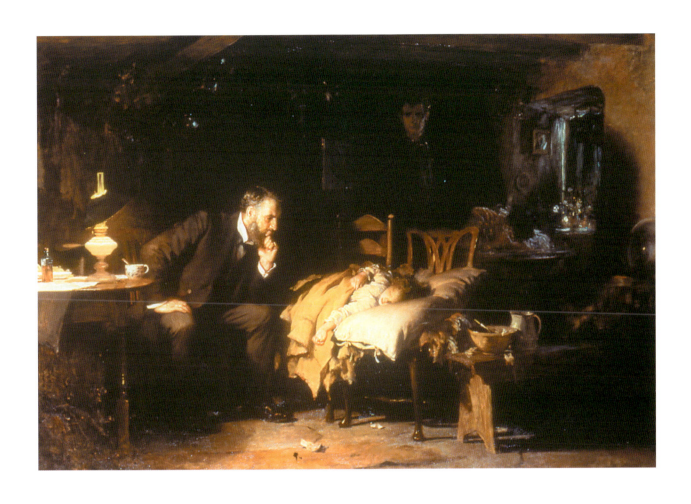

The Doctor (c 1891) by Sir Luke Fildes (© Tate, London 2002).

34

Doctor Teaching on a Sick Child Before an Audience of Doctors and Students, New York Polyclinic School of Medicine (1891)

by Irving R. Wiles

From the Renaissance onwards, in anatomy (witness Rembrandt's *Anatomy Lesson of Dr Tulp*) and to some extent in surgery, it was recognised that practical demonstrations were an important adjunct to formal lectures and learning from textbooks. Certainly by the 19th century teaching demonstrations with live patients had also become an important aspect of undergraduate and postgraduate teaching in medicine. The eliciting of the relevant medical history and the patient's symptoms followed by the demonstration of important clinical signs became the hallmark of medical teaching. This woodcut with added colour by the American artist and illustrator Irving Ramsey Wiles shows a typical teaching session in a paediatric clinic at the turn of the 19th century.

By then women were just beginning to be admitted to the profession and Wiles has included in his painting three females among the audience. There had been strong opposition to women entering the profession and they began by founding their own medical schools when excluded from existing ones. For instance in the United States the Women's Medical College of Philadelphia opened in 1850, and the Women's College of New York in 1865. In the UK the London School of Medicine for Women was opened in 1874. Among the women at the time who qualified in medicine were Elizabeth Blackwell in New York in 1849 and Elizabeth Garrett who obtained, by a legal loophole, a diploma of the Society of Apothecaries in London in 1865. But though allowed to study medicine, women were barred from the more prestigious schools of medicine until much later. For example women were not admitted to the University of Edinburgh Medical School until 1889 and to many of the London medical schools until after the First World War.

In this painting of the New York Polyclinic School of Medicine in 1891, the teacher, formally dressed but without the professional white coat, discusses the case of a sick infant. The mother stands demurely behind. Another mother with her infant waits on the left. Such case presentations, often in the form of so-called 'grand rounds', are now a major feature of clinical teaching in medical schools and other medical institutions.

The painter of this interesting work, Irving Ramsey Wiles (1861–1948), was the son of an artist and studied in New York under William Merritt Chase, famed for his portraiture. Wiles emulated his style and during the 1890s became himself a highly successful portrait painter with a magnificent studio in New York. This illustration is therefore not typical of his work, but to many it is of special interest in depicting a scene of clinical teaching which would become universally accepted over the years.

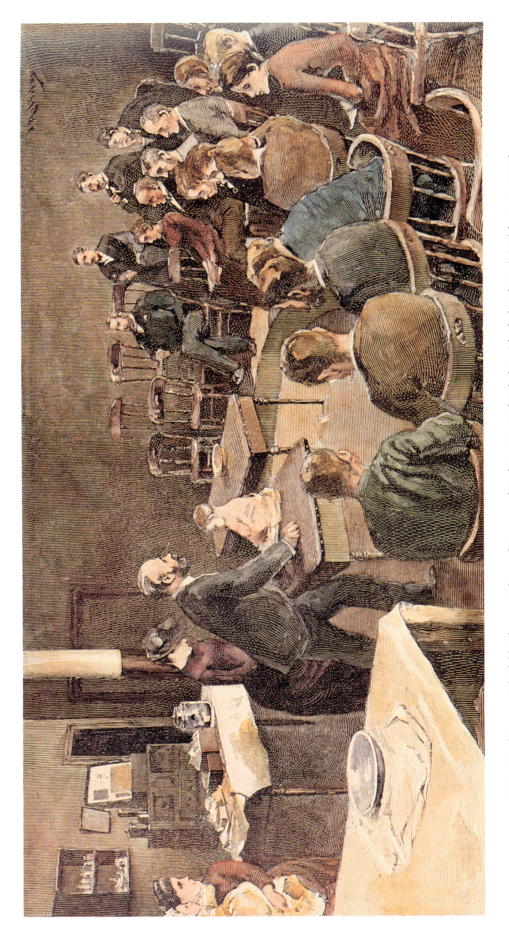

Doctor Teaching on a Sick Child Before an Audience of Doctors and Students, New York Polyclinic School of Medicine (1891) by Irving R. Wiles.

36

Science and Charity (1897)

by Pablo Picasso

The name Pablo Picasso (1881–1973) is usually associated with the Cubist movement which he originated at the beginning of the last century with his famous painting *Demoiselles d'Avignon* of 1907, where forms are broken down into planes. However this painting, *Science and Charity*, is one of his early works which gives no indication of how his art would develop in the following ten years.

Picasso was born in Malaga in 1881, the son of a conventional painter and art teacher at the local school of Fine Arts. His father, José Ruiz Blasco (Picasso used his mother's name), features in several of Picasso's early paintings, including this one. In 1897 at the age of 16 he went to study in Madrid for a short period but it was only later in Barcelona that his precocious and exceptional talent began to develop and show itself.

His father, being an artist himself, encouraged his son's talents from an early age. But he attempted to mould his son along his own lines of academic painting of country scenes, genre work and conventional portraiture. His father's influence in these directions is clearly evident in several of Picasso's early works. In this painting, *Science and Charity*, Picasso's father sat for the doctor. The model for the patient is unknown but the baby was borrowed from a beggar woman for the painting, and the nun's habit was also borrowed. The work suggests the skill and knowledge of a doctor. His habit of taking the patient's pulse and his serious manner imply that he provides the science involved in caring for the patient. The nun, seen here offering a drink and holding, one assumes, the patient's child, illustrates the caring aspect of medicine. The painting won Honourable Mention in Madrid, followed by a Gold Medal in Malaga and went to the house of Dr Salvador, Picasso's uncle. A very remarkable painting by a boy of only sixteen years of age.

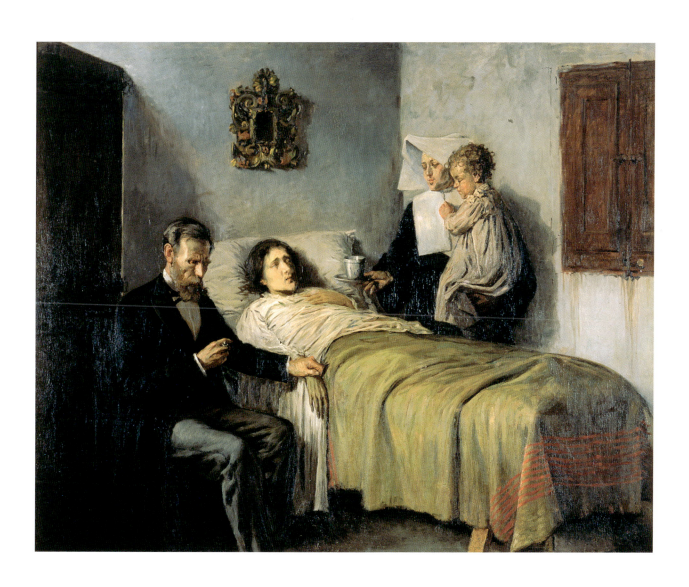

Science and Charity (1897) by Pablo Picasso (Museu Picasso, Barcelona, © Succession Picasso/DACS 2002. Photo supplied by Museu Picasso, Barcelona © Photo Arxiu Fotográphic de Museus, Ajuntament de Barcelona).

37

Le Tubage (1904)

by Georges Chicotot

There have been several surgeons who also became distinguished artists. They include such notables as Sir Charles Bell (1774–1842), Sir Francis Haden (1818–1910), Henry Tonks (1862–1937), a renowned war artist, Frank Netter (1906–1990) who illustrated Ciba Pharmaceutical material and of course, Sir Roy Calne (b 1930). There have however been very few practising physicians who at the same time became noted artists. One such was John Wells (1907–2000), a general practitioner in the Isles of Scilly where he built his own small hospital. He later became a full-time artist among the St Ives Group which at the time included Ben Nicholson and Barbara Hepworth to whom Wells became an assistant.

Georges-Alexandre Chicotot belongs to this rare group of practising physicians who also became accomplished artists. Unfortunately little is known of his personal life except that he was born in Paris. He first graduated from the École des Beaux-Arts in Paris and then later the École du Médicine from where he qualified in 1899. He subsequently became Head of Radiotherapy at the Hôpital Broca.

He first exhibited at the Salon in 1880. Many of his early works were of religious or historical subjects. But later in the early years of the twentieth century he began to concentrate on contemporary themes, often of a medical nature. Particularly noteworthy was his depiction in 1908 of an early attempt to treat cancer of the breast with X-rays in which the artist included a portrait of himself treating the patient.

In this painting a Doctor Albert Josias, a noted researcher of infectious diseases at the time, is surrounded by several doctors, one of whom is Chicotot himself, as he carries out an intubation on a child with croup. This is a syndrome characterised by stridor, cough and hoarseness due to airway obstruction. There are many causes but at the time this picture was painted a leading cause would have been diphtheria, where intubation or even tracheostomy can be life-saving. The artist has caught the intense involvement of all concerned in this life-saving procedure on a little child.

Chicotot received a number of awards during his lifetime, including a bronze medal at the World Exposition and later a Légion d'Honneur in 1922.

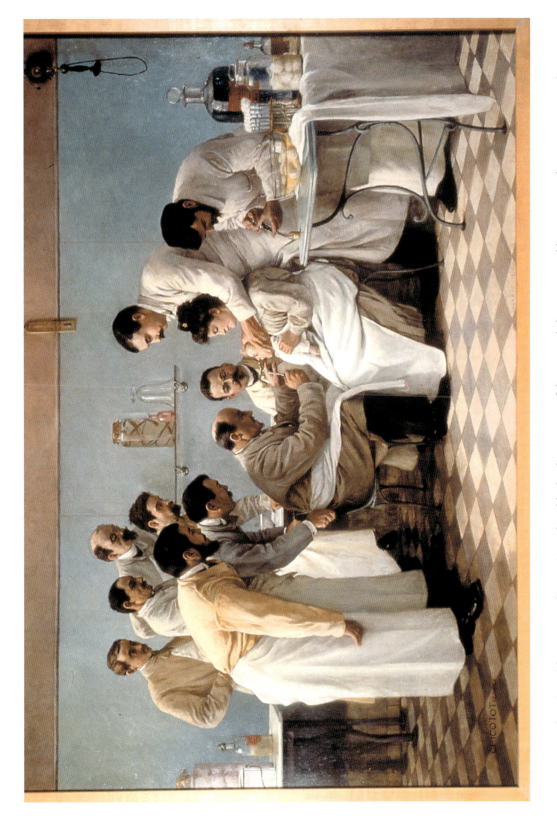

Le Tubage (1904) by Georges Chicotot (reproduced by kind permission of the *Musée de l'Assistance Publique*, Paris and SIPA Press, France).

38

Sentence of Death (1908)

by John Collier

There are few situations in the practice of medicine more traumatic than having to tell a patient that the problem is incurable and will be fatal. This painting by John Collier (1850–1934) is unique in depicting such an event. The sombre tones used by the artist help to emphasise the gravity of the situation. The patient sits uncomfortably, staring ahead, isolated in his grief. He sees no future. His facial pallor and demeanour contrast starkly with those of the doctor. The young man given the sentence of death was Gerald Layton Orr, a friend of the artist himself. When the painting was first exhibited there was much speculation about the possible nature of the terminal illness. This might have been a malignancy or perhaps an incurable infectious disease, since this was painted well before the advent of antibiotics. The microscope suggests perhaps its use for a sputum or blood test for tuberculosis or syphilis for example.

The painter himself, the Hon. John Collier, was the son of Judge Robert Collier (later first Lord Monkswell). He was educated at Eton and his original intention was to become a diplomat. He went abroad to study French and German and for a time worked as a clerk in the Foreign Office. But he then turned to painting and, with encouragement from Alma-Tadema and Millais, studied art at the Slade School under Edward Poynter. Eventually he established a successful society portrait practice. He married, in succession, two daughters of T.H. Huxley, the first of whom (Marian) was also a painter and died shortly after giving birth to their only child. He had a further son and daughter by his second wife. Collier exhibited on numerous occasions at the Royal Academy right until the year he died. His many portraits include those of Charles Darwin, T.H. Huxley, Ray Lankester, Kitchener, Bland-Sutton, Aldous Huxley and many others. But he also had a particular penchant for depicting psychological tragedies in modern life, such as *The Cheat* (1905), *Marriage de Convenance* (1907), *A Fallen Idol* (1913) and of course *Sentence of Death* (1908).

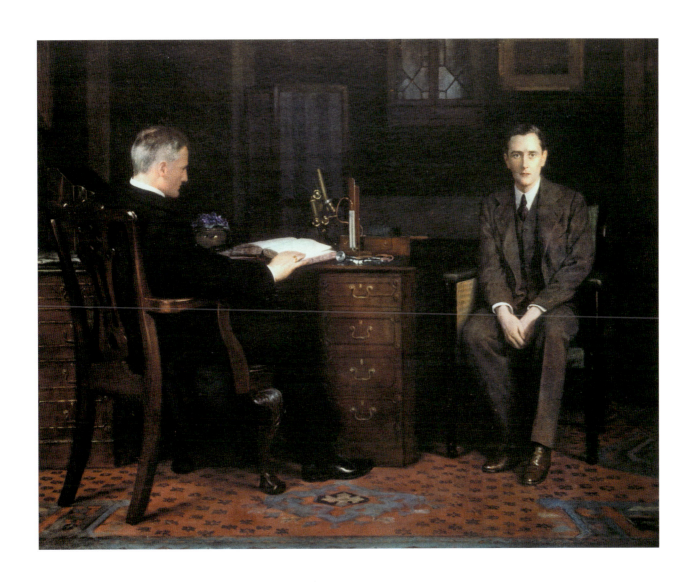

Sentence of Death (1908) by John Collier (reproduced by kind permission of the Wellcome Library, London and the Estate of John Collier).

39

The First Wounded, London Hospital 1914 (1915)

by John Lavery

This painting records an event which, like many of Lavery's paintings, were very popular at the time. Lavery (1856–1941) was born in Belfast but was orphaned in early childhood and Glasgow became his adopted home. Here he later studied at the Glasgow School of Art and subsequently in Paris. He became a leading member of a group of artists known as the 'Glasgow Boys'. His career took off following his depiction of Queen Victoria and other notables at the Glasgow International Exhibition in 1888 and shortly afterwards, with encouragement from Whistler, he moved to London. He became renowned for his society portraits and for recording notable occasions and was knighted in 1918 and became an RA in 1921.

Though not in the forefront of British artists of the period, Lavery is noteworthy for the meticulous detail with which he recorded events. Lavery's War pictures contain, as he saw it, '… new beauties of colour and design …', with an accent upon spontaneity. In this painting for instance, the details of the hospital ward at the time are minutely recorded. The large Union flag reminds the viewer of patriotism at a time when the first injured servicemen were returning to the United Kingdom. By the side of each patient's bed is a locker with a vase of flowers. A visitor sits reading a paper and smoking a pipe! Half-way along the ward a physician in his dark suit converses with a nurse about a patient seated in a wheelchair. There are railed curtains around each bed to create some privacy though they do not extend the length of the bed. The nurse in her starched uniform and traditional bonnet attends a wounded soldier whose identity tag is clearly visible. Many of the detailed arrangements in this large, multi-bedded ward were not to change significantly for several decades.

When first exhibited at the Royal Academy in 1915 an art critic at the time singled out the painting for special mention as a remarkable achievement in a difficult study of the effects of interior illumination. A photogravure of the painting was issued by the Fine Art Society in aid of the work of the hospital.

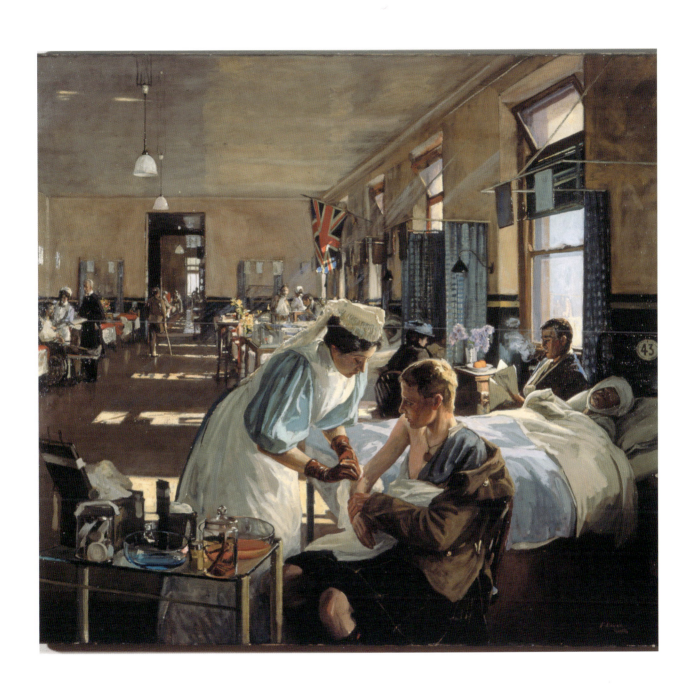

The First Wounded, London Hospital, 1914 (1915) by John Lavery (reproduced by kind permission of McManus Galleries, Dundee City Council Leisure and Arts).

40

An Advanced Dressing Station in France, 1918 (1918)

by Henry Tonks

Henry Tonks (1862–1937) first studied medicine at the London Hospital Medical College from 1881 to 1886, and subsequently became House Surgeon to Frederick Treves who encouraged Tonks' interest in surgery. In fact, he became a Fellow of the Royal College of Surgeons in 1888 and practised at the Royal Free Hospital. But his interest in art was obvious from an early age and later he chose art rather than surgery as his career. He studied the subject at the Westminster School under Frederick Brown and became his assistant at the Slade where Tonks later succeeded Brown as Slade Professor in 1918. His success as an artist included an exhibition of his work at the Tate Gallery in 1936. He had a dominant effect on English art in the first half of the last century, with his particular emphasis on drawing and draughtsmanship. Rex Whistler, Sir Stanley Spencer and Augustus John for example all trained under him.

In the First World War he held a commission in the RAMC and later was appointed an official war artist. In 1918 he produced this painting and commented at the time, 'The advanced dressing station was an incredible sight in time of battle, a kind of organised confusion, by this I mean an apparent confusion because they were beautifully run and I pride myself that it gives a reasonable account of modern war.' Here the surgeons and doctors are caring for those recently wounded. The carnage and suffering are depicted in a way that evokes great sympathy for the suffering soldiers and the humanity of those caring for them. Tonks drew and painted many other surgical and medical subjects of the war with collections now in the Imperial War Museum and the Victoria and Albert Museum in London.

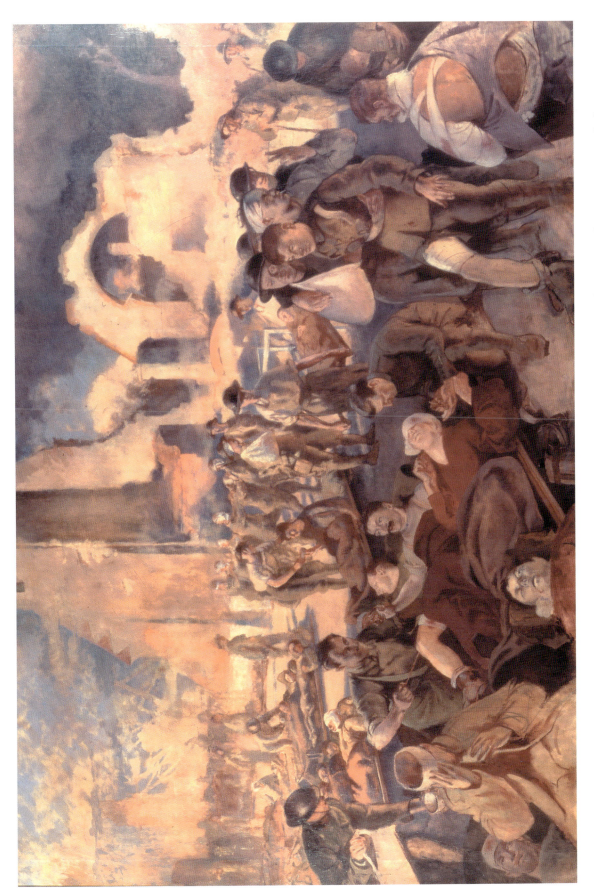

An Advanced Dressing Station in France, 1918 (1918) by Henry Tonks (reproduced by kind permission of The Imperial War Museum, London).

41

Bed Making (1932)

by Sir Stanley Spencer

Stanley Spencer (1891–1959) has been described by critics as one of the best-known and perhaps best-loved of all twentieth-century British artists. His popularity is based largely on his celebration of English parochial life in Cookham, a small community 25 miles west of London, where he spent a total of 49 of his 68 years. The main emphasis of his work was the depiction of biblical themes painted with simplicity and sincerity.

He had a rather unconventional upbringing and early education. Then in 1908 at the age of 17 he began to study at the Slade School in London where he soon demonstrated his skill in draughtsmanship. His painting *The Nativity* won first prize at the Slade Summer Exhibition. In 1915 he enlisted in the Royal Army Medical Corps and worked for a year as an orderly at Beaufort War Hospital near Bristol where he had first-hand experience of the devastating effects of war injuries. In 1916 he was posted to Macedonia where he served with the Field Ambulances and later as an infantryman, and returned to Cookham in December 1918. These experiences affected him greatly but it was not until 1923 that he planned a major series of works based on his memories of active service. Louis and Mary Behrend then commissioned a memorial to their friend's brother, Lieutenant Henry Willoughby Sandham, who had died on active service. They arranged to build a private chapel, the Sandham Chapel at Burghclere, to house a series of murals to be painted by Spencer which would include an altarpiece, *The Resurrection of the Soldiers*. He painted the Sandham Memorial Chapel in order to redeem his appalling wartime experiences by translating them into art. He commented himself, ' … that operation redeemed my experience from what it was; namely something alien to me. By this means I recover my lost self.'

One of the panels in the Chapel is entitled *Bed Making*. The patient on the left is asleep and snugly huddled in his blankets with a large hot-water bottle. Warmth and homeliness are also emphasised by the floral bed coverings, the photographs on the wall and the warmth of the electric light. This is an atmosphere much at variance with the wartime experiences of the wounded service men. It also emphasises the importance of orderlies and other ancillary ward staff. The important role that they can play in the care of the sick can too easily be neglected.

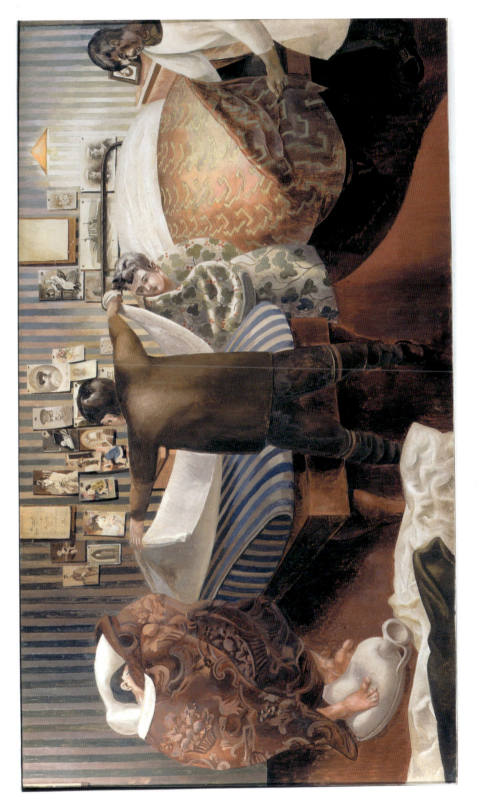

Bed Making (1932) by Sir Stanley Spencer. Sandham Memorial Chapel (National Trust) Burghclere. (© Estate of Stanley Spencer 2002. All Rights Reserved, DACS. Photo courtesy of National Trust Photographic Library).

42

Hospital Ward II (1920)

by Hilding Linnqvist

Hilding Linnqvist (1891–1984) was born in Stockholm and spent his working life in the city though he travelled widely in Europe and North Africa. In his early training he was much influenced by Edvard Munch and Ernst Josephson. He became a designer of stage sets, mosaics and tapestries, and as a painter, at least up to the 1950s, he was best known for his 'naïve' style. Painters of this school were trained artists who deliberately adopted a child-like, simplistic style. Later Linnqvist became increasingly influenced by Cézanne and his work lost its early naïve approach.

His earlier style is well-illustrated in *Hospital Ward II*. Though the picture is superficially simple, more careful study reveals that it is both complex and subtle. The doctors are portrayed as doll-like figures and they and the nurses attending the patient are completely out of proportion to the figures in the rest of the ward. They are almost puppet-like. The doctor on the left seems to be examining a specimen tube, the patient has closed eyes, and a relative (behind the doctor) is portrayed in black, perhaps grieving. The orderliness of the ward and the line-up of erect senior nursing figures give the impression of a rigid hierarchy. In contrast the postures of the junior nurses bending over and actually attending to the patients convey the impression of tenderness and that they are more involved in caring. It is quite reasonable that an outsider, rightly or wrongly, could gather such an impression of the various individuals on a hospital ward round.

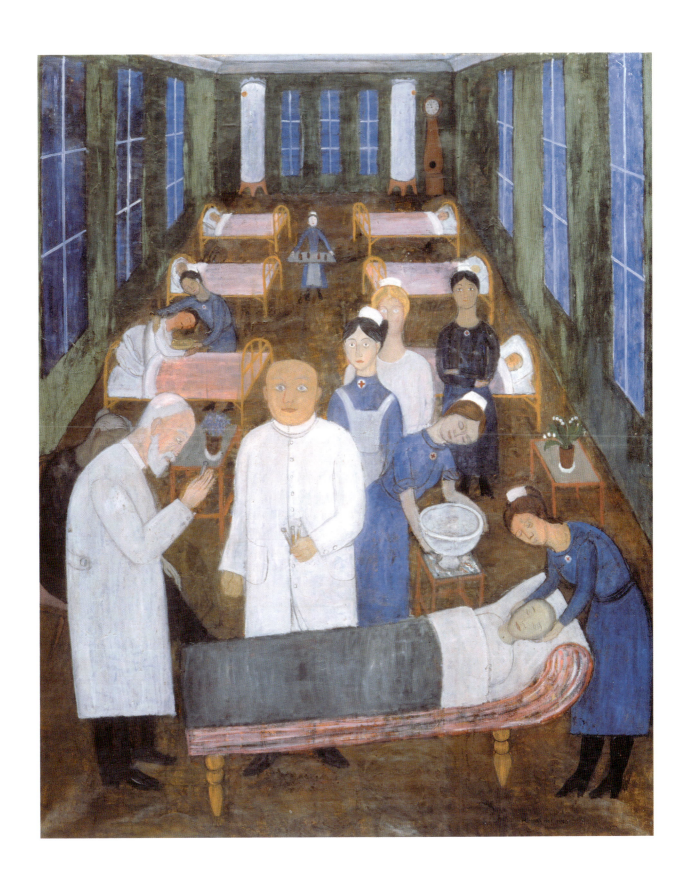

Hospital Ward II (1920) by Hilding Linnqvist (reproduced by kind permission of the Moderna Museet, Stockholm and ©DACS 2002).

44

Doctor and Doll (1929)

by Norman Rockwell

Norman Rockwell's paintings epitomised liberal, middle-class American society from the time of the First World War. He was born in New York in February 1894 and died in Stockbridge, Maine in November 1978. He studied at the Chase School of Fine and Applied Art, the National Academy of Art and the Art Students League in New York. Subsequently he studied in Paris for a time. Though an admirer of Picasso and other modernists he himself remained a realist American genre painter in a style similar to Winslow Homer (1836–1910) and Thomas Eakins (1844–1916). His early career was essentially as an illustrator for boys' magazines and later the *Encyclopaedia Britannica* but he was best known in America for his covers for the popular weekly magazine, the *Saturday Evening Post*, an association which lasted 47 years with more than 300 cover illustrations. Over the years he depicted many aspects of American life with warmth and humour, as in this painting. In World War II his famous 'Four Freedoms' posters were much acclaimed and included for example his *Freedom of Speech* (now in the Metropolitan Museum of Art). Presidents Eisenhower, Kennedy and Johnson all sat for him in portraits, and he also painted Colonel Nasser of Egypt and Prime Minister Nehru of India. After the war he turned his attention to problems of racial segregation, the Peace Corps volunteers and similar issues. In 1957 the US Chamber of Commerce cited him as a Great Living American by concluding that 'Through the magic of your talent, the folks next door – their gentle sorrows, their modest joys – have enriched our own lives and given us new insight into our countrymen.'

Until recently his work has not always found favour with the great art galleries, perhaps because he was often considered more an illustrator than an artist. But this may be changing following a major retrospective in New York in 2002. *Doctor and Doll* is very typical of Rockwell's art. The family doctor attempts to win the trust of his little patient by pretending to examine her doll. The expression on the doctor's face is very convincing, though the little girl still seems somewhat apprehensive. But how many doctors have resorted to such a ruse, and still do, to win the trust of their young patients? The certificate above the doctor's desk indicates his Registration in the state of Vermont and his work chair, doctor's bag and even his dress all suggest a family practitioner. His career has been his life. The arrangement of the well-worn books and candlesticks almost resembles an altar. Everything in Rockwell's picture conjures up the image of a careful, kind and much-loved and respected family doctor.

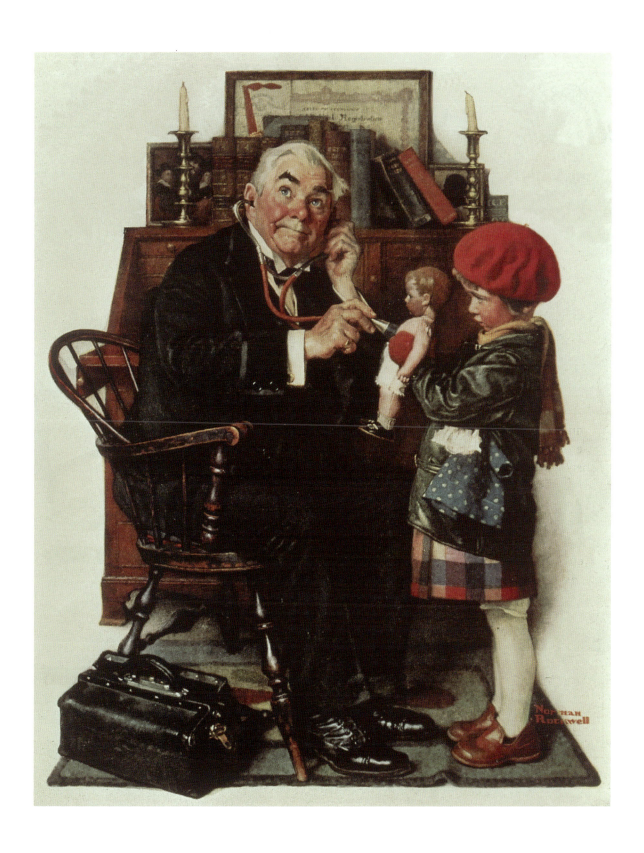

Doctor and Doll (1929) by Norman Rockwell (reproduced by kind permission of the Norman Rockwell Family Agency; © the Norman Rockwell Entities).

45

Norman Rockwell Visits a Family Doctor (1947)

by Norman Rockwell

Norman Rockwell's (1894–1978) background as an artist and realist American genre painter has already been described. It is therefore interesting to compare the previous painting *Doctor and Doll* (1929) with this later painting. Both depict the relationship between doctor and patient, but are treated very differently. In *Doctor and Doll*, we see the caring family doctor who has clearly been practising for many years and knows how to win over the confidence of his little patient. But then there was very little at the time the doctor could do in the way of investigation or treatment of many childhood diseases, such as scarlet fever and diphtheria. The doctor's role was therefore often limited essentially to sympathetic caring.

Following the Second World War however, matters began to change particularly with improved and more accessible means of investigation and the advent of better treatments, most notably following the introduction of penicillin and streptomycin.

In this picture of 1947 the image is still that of a caring family doctor here surrounded by suggestions of a possible rural practice: the stag's head and shotgun over the fireplace and the border collie sitting on a rocking chair by the fire. Rockwell in fact was living in rural Vermont at the time. But the many books on the doctor's shelves imply his greater learning. The contrivance on the right is possibly X-ray equipment, which is now rarely seen in a doctor's office, but here emphasises the technology being introduced into medicine as does the lamp on the left, which suggests other devices to aid the examination and investigation of his patients. He now also has a telephone. But his stethoscope still remains important. Concern is reflected in the doctor's face, cleverly highlighted by the reading lamp on the desk, and judging by the concentrated attention of the mother and father he clearly retains their respect – perhaps more than ever before.

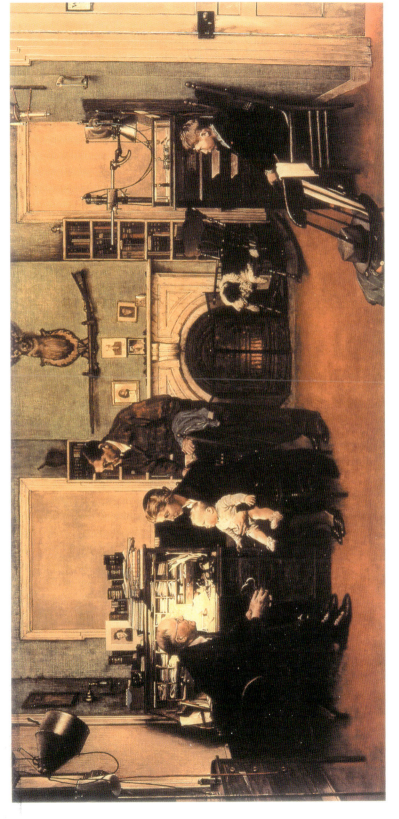

Norman Rockwell Visits a Family Doctor (1947) by Norman Rockwell (reproduced by kind permission of the Norman Rockwell Family Agency; © the Norman Rockwell Entities).

46

Children's Doctor (1949)

by Andrew Wyeth

Johns Hopkins Hospital and School of Medicine in Baltimore was founded in 1889 with four legendary figures: Osler (physician), Welch (pathologist), Halsted (surgeon) and Kelly (gynaecologist) who were largely responsible for ensuring the School would prosper and become one of the leading medical institutions in the world. But it almost failed early on through a budget deficit of some $500,000 needed for completion. A group of four young women however came to the rescue, one of whom was Mary Elizabeth Garrett, a very wealthy Baltimore philanthropist and daughter of Robert W. Garrett, president of the Baltimore & Ohio Railroad. They agreed to provide the necessary funds but on the condition that the school would admit women. The authorities were forced to agree and the School opened as a co-educational institution in 1893. Of the twenty members of the original class, three were women.

Dr Margaret Handy (1889–1977), the subject of this painting, graduated from Johns Hopkins in 1916 at the age of 27 and was one of the first to specialise in Paediatrics. She settled in Wilmington, Delaware where, at the time the picture was painted, she was the only woman out of six certified paediatricians.

The painter Andrew Wyeth (b. 1917) comes from a line of American artists which included his father (N.C. Wyeth, 1882–1945), an illustrator of children's books, and his son (James Wyeth, b. 1946), noted for his portraits which include those of John F. Kennedy and Andy Warhol. Andrew Wyeth is perhaps best known for his scenes of rural American life mainly around his home at Chadds Ford, Pennsylvania. In 1949 the artist's young son, Nicholas, became very ill and Margaret Handy cared for him, driving out to their house at any time of the day or night. The boy recovered and in this painting the artist has captured the thoughtful concerned expression of the doctor with just a hint of weariness. She is also seen striding away in the moon-light to another patient. A fond tribute to a caring and hard-working children's doctor.

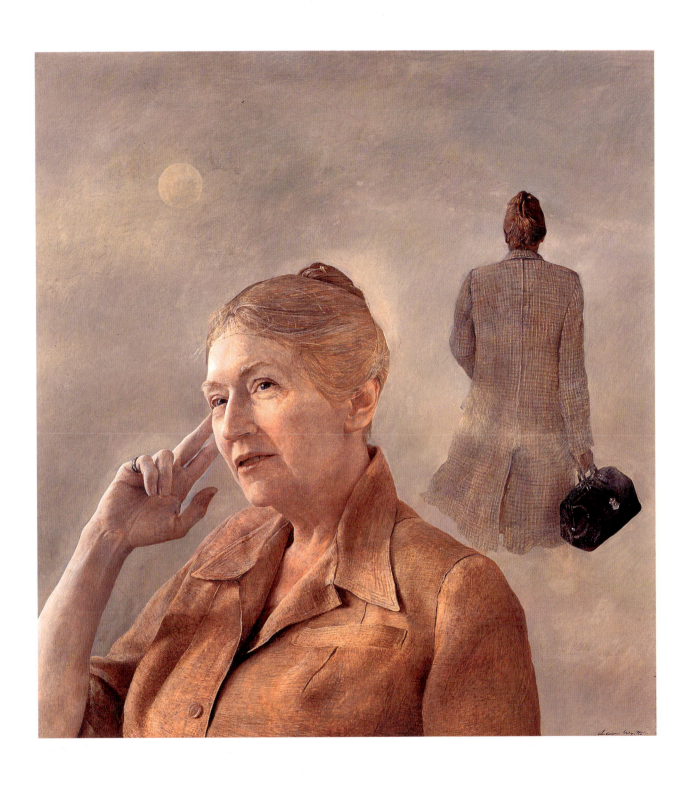

Children's Doctor (1949) by Andrew Wyeth, (reproduced by kind permission of the Brandywine River Museum, Chadds Ford, Pennsylvania. Gift of Betsy James Wyeth (artist's wife), © Andrew Wyeth).

47

The Doctor (1950)

by Anna Mary Robertson Moses ('Grandma Moses')

Though a work of 1950, this painting of an American farmstead is evocative of a bygone age. Horses graze in a distant field and children are playing in the foreground. The doctor, carrying his bag, has arrived on horseback on a domiciliary visit presumably at the request of the farmer, perhaps to see one of the children. His attire and that of the lady by his side is of a previous age.

The artist was a very remarkable woman. Grandma Moses is a pseudonym for Anna Mary Moses (née Robertson) who was born in 1860 in Greenwich, New York of Scots–Irish descent, and died in Hoosick Falls, New York in 1961 at the age of 101. She was the third of ten children and worked on a neighbouring farm from the age of 12 until she married Thomas Salmon Moses in 1887. The couple went on later to farm in Eagle Bridge, New York.

She had been encouraged by her father to draw and paint, but busy farm life left her little time for more than occasional decorative work and embroidery which became increasingly difficult with arthritis in later life. So she turned to painting only in the 1930s when already in her 70s. In 1938 some of her work was hung in a local drug store and this caught the attention of a collector and led to her being 'discovered'. With encouragement she went on to have a one-man show in New York in 1940 at the age of 80. This was an immediate success and a review in the New York Herald Tribune referred to her as 'Grandma Moses', a name by which she is now known in the art world.

She enjoyed increasing public acclaim and became a celebrity. In 1949 she was received at the White House by President Harry Truman, in 1955 commissioned to paint President Eisenhower's farm and in 1960 Governor Nelson Rockefeller proclaimed her birthday (September 7) as 'Grandma Moses Day' in New York State.

Her paintings, mainly on board and widely reproduced on greetings cards, fabrics and wallpapers, are generally of rural scenes redolent of a past time of serene country life. This painting of a country doctor's visit is typical.

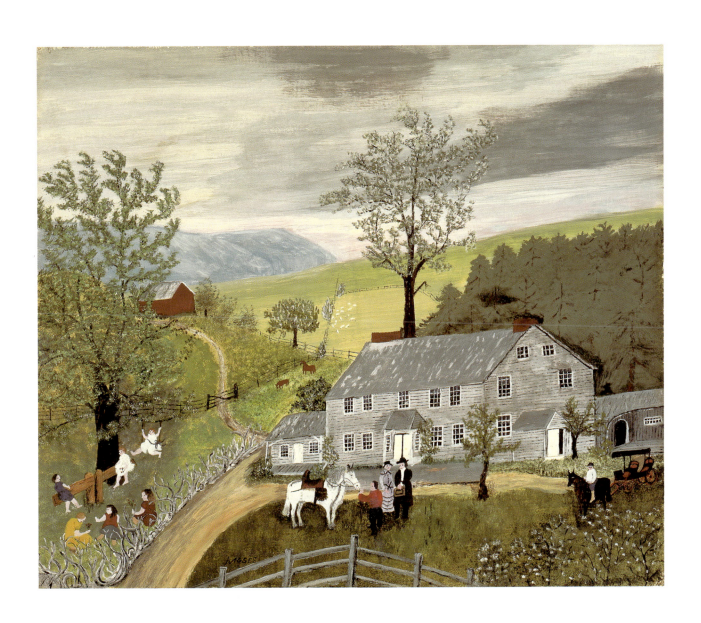

Grandma Moses: *The Doctor*. Copyright © 1951 (renewed 1979) Grandma Moses Properties Co., New York.

48

Ancoats Hospital Outpatients' Hall (1952)

by L.S. Lowry

Laurence Stephen Lowry was born in 1887 in Manchester and spent his entire life in and around the city. He never married and lived with his parents until they died. For 42 years he was a rent collector with the same company. From early on however, he attended evening classes in art, first at the Municipal College of Art in Manchester and later at the Salford School of Art. His early paintings of still lifes, landscapes and portraits (most notably of himself and his mother) were certainly accomplished. But it was his depictions of industrial working class scenes of Lancashire for which he is best remembered. The scene of a hospital outpatient hall in the early 1950s is all too evocative. Patients sat in long rows, moving up one at a time as their names were called from one of the consulting rooms at the back of the hall. Patients and relatives often struck up friendships with others while waiting and shared details of their complaints and treatments. It was the early days of the NHS, antibiotics were now becoming available and there was an optimism among both patients and doctors for the future of modern medicine. However not everyone in this painting seems to share this optimism!

Lowry himself was always self-deprecating about his art but to many he provided a unique insight into the people and places of an era which has passed. It was only late in his career that his work began really to be appreciated. He died after a short illness in February 1976 at the age of 88, just a few months before a major retrospective exhibition of 300 of his works was to be held at the Royal Academy.

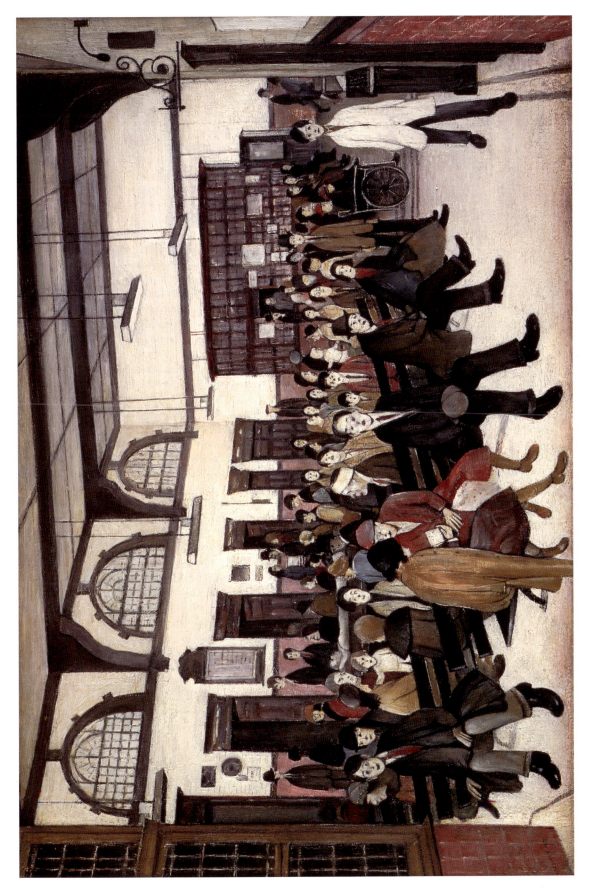

Ancoats Hospital Outpatients' Hall (1952) by L.S. Lowry (reproduced by kind permission of Carol A Lowry, the copyright holder. Image supplied by the Whitworth Art Gallery, University of Manchester, UK).

49

Healing of a Lunatic Boy (1986)

by Stephen Conroy

Certain Christian sects, most notably Christian Scientists, view sickness and recovery as being entirely due to the intervention of Providence and God's will. Sin was considered the cause of illness and could therefore be healed by prayer. This approach to disease goes back a long way to the teachings of the Bible. Even today faith healing still has a large following, highlighted for example by certain television evangelists in the United States. Often this takes the form of prayer with the 'laying-on of hands.'

Faith healing in a present-day setting is illustrated in this painting by Stephen Conroy. The artist was born in 1964 in Helensburgh, Scotland and studied art at the Glasgow School of Art, and in 1986 he was awarded First Prize for painting at the Royal Academy. He plans his paintings meticulously with detailed drawings. Commentators have noted his frequent use of chiaroscuro with strong contrasts of light and shade, in order to create dramatic effects. Furthermore in this picture the artist has compressed his subjects into a shallow picture space with little apparent communication between them, thus emphasising a claustrophobic atmosphere. The healer is imploring Providence to effect a cure, praying aloud with his eyes closed and his arm outstretched in supplication. His attendants also appear to be praying. But the deathly pallor of the sick boy suggests that faith healing seems unlikely to be effective.

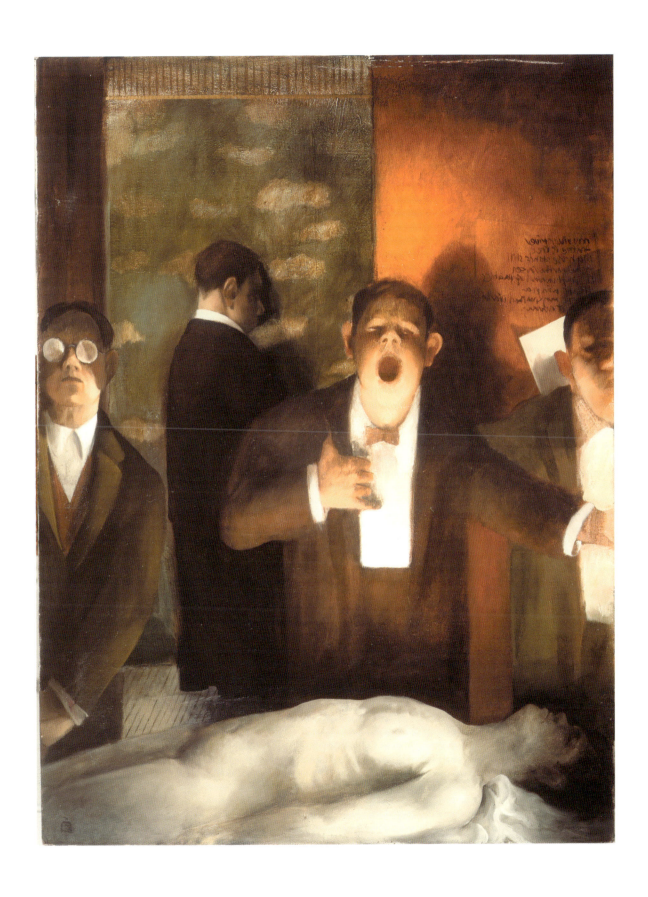

The Healing of a Lunatic Boy (1986) by Stephen Conroy (Scottish National Gallery of Modern Art, Edinburgh).

50

The Madhouse (1987)

by Sergei Chepik

Until about 40 years ago the long-term care of the mentally ill in Britain was mainly consigned to large mental institutions or asylums. But it became clear with the advent of new effective treatments, such as lithium for manic depression in 1949 followed by other anti-depressants and anti-psychotics in the early 1950s, that the care of the less severely affected and treatable cases could be transferred to the community. This large painting by the Russian-born artist Sergei Chepik reminds the viewer of the darker side of asylum life and has captured the dismal and depressing atmosphere of some of these institutions. The fabric of the building is clearly in a bad state of repair and the inmates are poorly cared for. The asylum was actually located in an old abandoned church with faded frescoes on the walls and as the artist comments, it had replaced a house of hope and prayer. In the background one inmate is bedridden and the remainder are all lost in their own thoughts. A group seated around a table seem to be occupied in a sort of discussion. According to the artist's comments on the work, in the USSR in those days '. . . lunatics, psychologically disturbed people and criminals as well as maniacs, neurotics and schizophrenics, drug addicts and potential suicide victims all shared the same institution'.

Chepik was born in Kiev in 1953, the year of Stalin's death, and came from a family of artists and academics. His grandparents befriended many distinguished artists and writers including Mikhail Bulgakov (1891–1940), a physician who qualified in medicine at Kiev University in 1916 but gave up practice in 1920 in order to devote himself entirely to writing but whose work was censured during the Stalinist era. To many he is well known for his *A Country Doctor's Notebook*, a down-to-earth and realistic description of his experiences as a doctor working under appalling conditions in a rural practice at the time.

Chepik trained at the Kiev Institute and later at the Repin Art Institute in Leningrad (now St Petersburg) where he graduated in 1978. He rapidly became known for his work and exhibited widely in the Soviet Union and also Japan. However he refused to accept Soviet ideology which he increasingly criticised in his work. In 1979 a doctor friend invited Chepik to come to his psychiatric institution in the hope of studying the effects of the artist's activity on the behaviour of his patients. Over a period of several months Chepik made many drawings and a year later returned to do a number of monotypes of the inmates. In the final painting, based on his studies and completed in 1987, Chepik has included himself sitting in the background near a window where he is observing and sketching the inmates. *The Madhouse* however was banned from being exhibited and the following year in 1988 Chepik left the Soviet Union to settle in Paris, where he now has a studio in Montmartre. The painting was acclaimed in France and later awarded a gold medal at the Salon d'Automne in Paris and has been described in detail in his wife's book on this very talented and original Russian painter (*Sergei Chepik*, by Marie-Aude Albert, Paris, 1994).

Chepik admits that the work is not only a depiction of a Russian mental asylum at the time but is also '. . . an allegorical representation of Soviet society, walled in by its own lies, paranoia and despair'. Somewhat appropriately the artist also entitled the painting *The House of the Dead*, redolent of Dostoyevsky's masterpiece *Memoirs from the House of the Dead*, written in 1862.

100

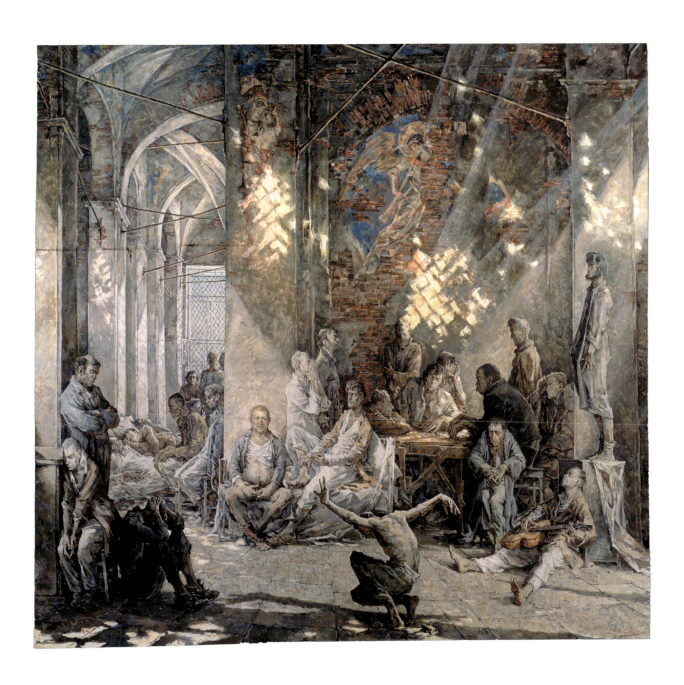

The Madhouse (1987) by Sergei Chepik (Private collection, London).

51

The Compassion of the Intensive Care Sister (1989)

by Sir Roy Calne

Very few individuals have become distinguished both as a physician or surgeon as well as a renowned artist. Sir Roy Calne (b. 1930) is such an individual. Until retirement he was Professor of Surgery at the University of Cambridge and was one of the major pioneers in transplant surgery. In fact he carried out the first human liver transplant outside the United States in 1968, some ten years after becoming a Fellow of the Royal College of Surgeons, London. Since then he and his team have performed over a thousand such operations with a high success rate. For his work he has received numerous awards and honours and he was elected a Fellow of the Royal Society in 1974, and knighted in 1986.

He has been painting from childhood but a turning point came when in 1988 he met the Scottish artist, John Bellany, who was then desperately ill and dying of liver disease. Following a successful liver transplant, Bellany stimulated Calne in his artistic endeavours and encouraged him to loosen his style and use brighter, vivid colours. This help and advice had a dramatic effect on Calne's style, as he admits: 'I started to think of painting as a means of emotional expression as opposed to merely producing an attractive picture'. This is well illustrated in this painting, one of Calne's most sensitive works. The post-operative care of the patient is extremely demanding and here he captures the attentive concern of the nursing sister at this critical period of the patient's recovery. He also incorporated a miniature of this same painting in his diptych *Homage to Mantegna and Saints Cosmas and Damian* (1990) in which he traces the events following a fatal motorcycle accident of the liver donor, an ambulance carrying the victim away, the grieving relatives, a helicopter transporting the donor organ, and the liver transplantation operation. By also including a miniature version of this painting of the compassionate nursing sister, Calne emphasised the heart-warming caring qualities of the team. It can be seen as epitomising his deeply felt regard for human life and the contribution of all those who strive in their various ways to preserve it.

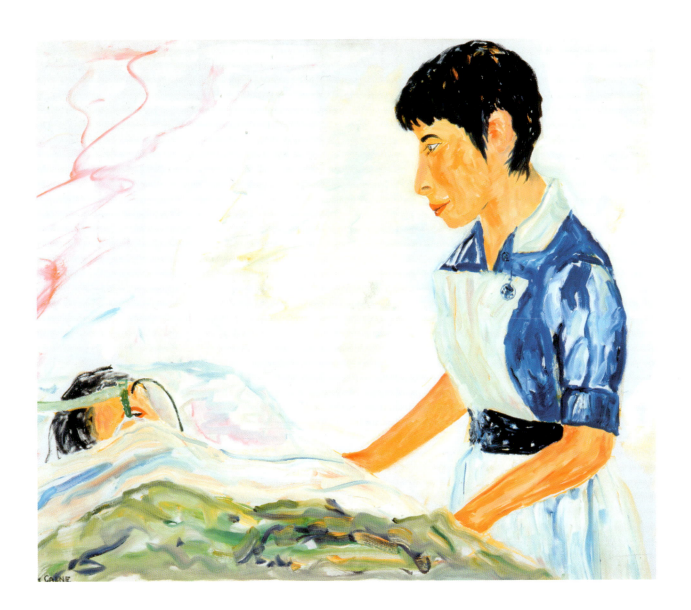

The Compassion of the Intensive Care Sister (1989) by Sir Roy Calne (reproduced by kind permission of the artist).

52

An African Healer Throwing Bones (2000)

by Meg Campbell

We have thus far been concerned primarily with the medical consultation as practised in Western art. But of course there are many societies which employ other approaches, and this is well exemplified in the case of divination by 'throwing bones' as practised by traditional healers in rural Africa. The coloured etching of a healer in her traditional red costume shows how she is attempting to assess the patient's likely outcome or prognosis from the arrangement of the bones she throws on the ground. Such healers often share the same culture, beliefs and values as their patients and in this way often have a profound understanding of their clients. At one time they were considered merely 'witch doctors' or shamans. But this ignores the close association and knowledge they have of the community. For this reason they can in fact become valuable partners in the delivery of health care in many rural communities.

Meg Campbell is a professional etcher and printmaker who has spent a great deal of her time with traditional healers. She was trained at the University of Witwatersrand in South Africa and at the West Surrey College of Art and Design. She has a particular interest in women's lives, centred on the theme of mother and child, and was an artist-in-residence at the Princess Anne Maternity Hospital in Southampton where she now lives. It was while holding a Churchill Travelling Fellowship in 1992 that she met Merci Mansi, a traditional healer who practised in a squatter settlement outside Johannesburg and was part of a group practice which used both traditional African and Western therapeutic methods. The present picture was made for the cover of the recent *Lancet Supplement 2000* 'One World, Many Voices'.

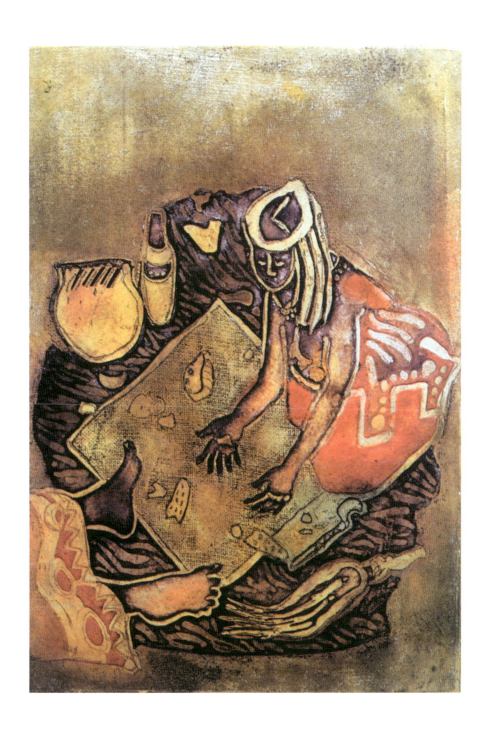

An African Healer Throwing Bones (2000) by Meg Campbell (reproduced by kind permission of the artist and *The Lancet* 356: s1:1).

53

The Patient and Researcher (2001)

by Louise Riley

Advances in medical science, particularly in more recent times, have led to the elucidation of the causes of many diseases and to finding effective treatments and even cures. But there still remain many conditions where the cause remains unknown and therapy is still limited. The more obvious examples are certain forms of cancer. The common multi-factorial disorders, also known as disorders of complex inheritance, are each due to several genes for susceptibility plus the effects of environmental factors. They include for example many neurological conditions, most notably multiple sclerosis and motor neurone disease, as well as certain psychiatric disorders such as schizophrenia. But though scientists are now beginning to identify some of the genes responsible for these conditions, the nature of any environmental factors remains largely unknown. In many inherited rare unifactorial disorders, the basic genetic defects have now been identified, thus making prevention possible through genetic counselling with prenatal diagnosis. But in order to find rational pharmacological treatments for these diseases it is also important to realise that the pathophysiology of most of these disorders still remains far from clear. As an alternative to drug treatment, attention is also being given to the possibilities of some form of effective gene or stem cell therapy.

There are therefore many gaps in our knowledge of the causes and possible treatment of many diseases and answers can only come through scientific research. The result is that in many cases, patients themselves often become the subject of such research by providing tissues for laboratory studies.

This illustration is actually an embroidery in which the London-based artist Louise Riley (b. 1981) has attempted to link the patient and researcher using the metaphor of puzzle pieces. In discussing her work she has written, 'My aim was to describe the physical aspect of the removal of organs and blood samples from the patient, and their redirection to a laboratory where a researcher would experiment, attempting to ascertain a diagnosis or cure – putting the puzzle pieces back together.'

The illustration was used by the journal *The Lancet* for the front cover of a supplement published in December 2001 which dealt with 33 diseases ranging from Alzheimer's disease to systemic lupus erythematosus. To quote from the editors of the supplement, 'We asked 33 doctors and scientists to explain what is exciting in their area of medicine [research] right now and we asked 33 individuals with first hand experience of the same diseases to write about their experience of it. We need to still get excited about what medicine and science can do, but we must also understand the priorities of those who have to live with illness.' So whatever the importance of medical research, the role of the practising physician should always be based on care and compassion, an ideal which we hope will remain unchanged in future.

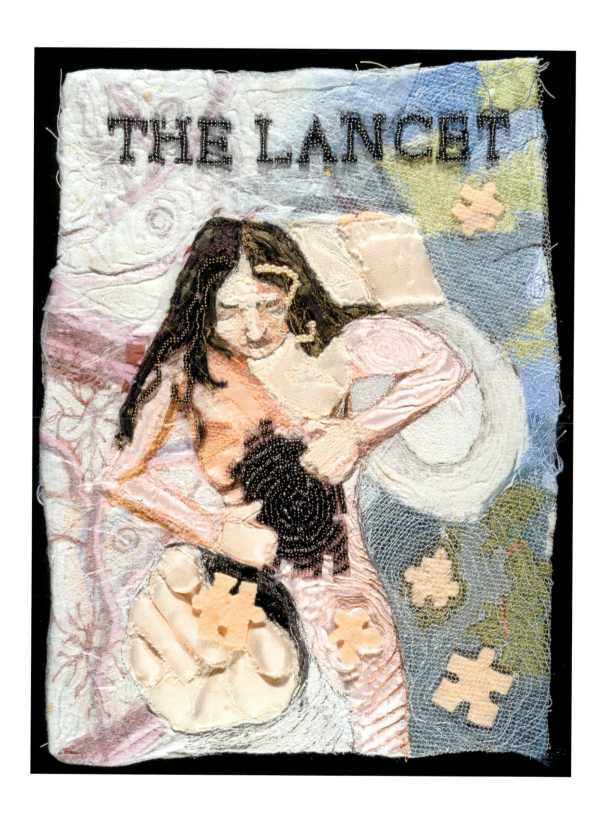

The Patient and the Researcher (2001) by Louise Riley (reproduced by kind permission of the artist and *The Lancet*).

A Selection of Medical Conditions Depicted in Paintings

DISORDER	PAINTING Title (date)	Location	ARTIST
Albinism	*Nude Girl on a Fur* (1932)	National Gallery of Modern Art, Edinburgh	Otto Dix (1891–1969)
Blindness	*Parable of the Blind* (1568)	Museo Nazionali, Naples	Pieter Brueghel (c 1525–1569)
	The Blind Man of Gambazo or *The Sense of Touch* (1632)	Prado, Madrid	Jusepe de Ribera (1591–1652)
	A Wedding Morning (c 1892)	Lever Art Gallery, Port Sunlight	John Henry Frederick Bacon (c 1866–1914)
Cleft lip	*Boy with Cleft Lip* (1902)	Tretiakov Gallery, Moscow	Mikhail Vrubel (1856–1910)
Clubfoot (*see also* **Hemiplegia**)	*Feeding the Hungry* (1504) (from the *Altarpiece of the Seven Works of Mercy*)	Rijksmuseum, Amsterdam	Master of Alkmaar (active 1490–1520)
Congenital heart disease (possibly Fallot's tetralogy)	*Various self-portraits*	Gemeentemuseum, Arnhem	Dick Ket (1902–1940)
Craniosynostosis (possibly Crouzon's disease)	*Count N. D. Guriev* (1821)	Hermitage, St. Petersburg	Jean-Auguste-Dominique Ingres (1780–1867)
Digital abnormalities			
• **Absent digit**	*Ernest Reinhold* (1908)	Musée des Beaux-Arts, Brussels	Oskar Kokoshka (1886–1980)
• **Polydactyly**	*Marriage of the Virgin* (1504)	Pinacoteca of Brera, Milan	Raphael (1483–1520)
	The Beautiful Gardener (1507–1508)	Louvre, Paris	Raphael (1483–1520)
	Self Portrait (1912)	Stedelijk Museum, Amsterdam	Marc Chagall (1887–1985)
• **Syndactyly**	*Portrait of a Canon* [identified as Nicolai Aegidius] (1517)	Royal Museum of Arts, Antwerp	Quentin Massys (c 1465–1530)
• **Thumb deformity**	*Erasmus* (1517)	Galleria Nazionale d'Arte Antica, Rome	Quentin Massys (c 1465–1530)
Down's syndrome (possibly)	*Adoration of the Shepherds* (c 1617)	Grenoble Museum	Jacob Jordaens (1593–1678)
	The Peasant and the Satyr (c 1638)	Staatliche Kunstsammlungen, Kassel	Jacob Jordaens (1593–1678)
	A Child with Nondisjunction (n.d.)	Private collection	Josef Warkany (1902–1992)
Duchenne muscular dystrophy (possibly)	*The Transfiguration* (1520)	Vatican Museum, Rome	Raphael (1483–1520)
	Sick Boy (1915)	Formerly Städtische Kunstsammlung Chemnitz, Karl-Marx-Stadt, Germany	Karl Schmidt-Rottluff (1884–1976)
Dupuytren's contracture	*Portrait of Fridel Battenberg* (1920)	Sprengel Museum, Hanover	Max Beckmann (1884–1950)
Dwarfism			
• **Disproportionate short stature**			
◇ **Achondroplasia**	*The Court Scene* from fresco, Camera degli Sposi (1474)	Palazzo Ducale, Mantua	Andrea Mantegna (c 1431–1506)
	Arrival of the English Ambassadors (1495–1500)	Accademia, Venice	Vittore Carpaccio (c 1465–1526)
	The Dwarf Morgante (c 1552)	Deposita della Soprintendenza, Florence	Angelo di Cosimo Bronzino (1503–1572)
	Moses Saved from the Waters (n.d.)	Pinacoteca of Brera, Milan	Bonifazio Veronese de Pitati (c 1487–1553)
	The Family of Darius before Alexander (c 1570)	National Gallery, London	Paolo Veronese (c 1528–1588)
	The Finding of Moses (1570–1580)	Prado, Madrid	Paolo Veronese (c 1528–1588)
	Arrigo peloso, Pietro matt and Amon nano (c 1598–1600)	Museo Nazionali di Capodimonte, Naples	Agostino Carraci (1557–1602)
	Apollo Killing the Cyclops (1616–1618)	National Gallery, London	Domenichino (Domenico Zampieri) (1581–1641)
	Artist's Studio (n.d.)	Bode Museum, Berlin	Jan Miense Molenaer (c 1610–1668)
	Don Baltasar Carlos with a Dwarf (1631–1632)	Isabella Stewart Gardner Museum, Boston	Velázquez (1599–1660)
	Peter's Denial of Christ (1636)	Szépmuvészeti Múzeum, Budapest	Jan Miense Molenaer (c 1610–1668)

DISORDER	PAINTING Title (date)	Location	ARTIST
	Calabazas (1637–1639)	Prado, Madrid	Velázquez (1599–1660)
	Las Meninas (1656)	Prado, Madrid	Velázquez (1599–1660)
	Il Cavadenti (c 1730)	Pinacoteca of Brera, Milan	Pietro Longhi (1702–1785)
	Francesco Ravai called Bajocco (1773)	Kunstmuseum, Copenhagen	Jens Juel (1745–1802)
	Grimaces et misères (1888)	Musée du Petit Palais, Paris	Fernand Pelez (1843–1913)
	The Dwarf Doña Mercedes (1899)	Musée d'Orsay, Paris	Ignacio Zuloaga (1870–1945)
◇ Diastrophic	*Sebastián de Morra* (c 1644–1651)	Prado, Madrid	Velázquez (1599–1660)
◇ Pseudo-achondroplasia	*El Primo* (1644)	Prado, Madrid	Velázquez (1599–1660)
	The Heidelberg Court Dwarf Perkeo (c 1730)	Kurpfälzisches Museum, Heidelberg	Johann Georg Dathan (1703–c 1764)
◇ Spondylo-epiphyseal dysplasia (possibly)	*Isabella Clara Eugenia with her Dwarf* (c 1580)	Prado, Madrid	Teodoro Felipe de Liaño (c 1515–1590)
	Aragonese Dwarf (1825)	Fogg Art Museum, Cambridge, Massachusetts	Vicente Lopez-y-Portana (1772–1850)
	Achille Emperaire (1820–1898) Aixois Painter (c 1868)	Musée d'Orsay, Paris	Paul Cézanne (1839–1906)
• **Proportionate short stature (pituitary)**	*Adoration of the Kings* (c 1472)	National Gallery, London	Sandro Botticelli (1445–1510)
	The Rich Epicure (n.d.)	Accademia, Venice	Bonifazio Veronese de Pitati (c 1487–1553)
	Cardinal Granvella's Dwarf and Dog (c 1560)	Louvre, Paris	Anthonis van Dashorst (called Antonio Moro) (1519–1575)
	Court Dwarf Estevanillo (1563–1568)	Staatliche Kunstsammlungen, Kassel	Anthonis van Dashorst (called Antonio Moro) (1519–1575)
	Festival in Honour of the Truce of 1609 (1616)	Louvre, Paris	Adriaen van de Venne (1589–1662)
	Philip IV and the Dwarf Soplillo (c 1618)	Prado, Madrid	Rodrigo de Villandrando (d. 1622)
	Aletheia Talbot and her Train (c 1630)	Alte Pinakothek, Munich	Peter Paul Rubens (1577–1640)
	Queen Henrietta and her Dwarf Sir Jeffrey Hudson (c 1633)	National Gallery, Washington, D.C.	Anthony van Dyck (1599–1641)
	King Charles II of Spain Attending an Auto-da-fé Accompanied by his Three Dwarfs (1680)	Prado, Madrid	Francisco Rizi (1608–1685)
	Portrait of the Court Dwarfess Mlle. Marichen (1684–1715)	Nationalhistoriske Museum pa Fredericksborg, Hillerød, Denmark	Jaques d'Agar (1640–1715)
	The Miniaturist Andreas von Behn (1700)	Gripsholm Palace, Swedish National Portrait Gallery, Stockholm	David von Krafft (1655–1724)
	The Salzburg Court Dwarf Franz von Meichelböck (c 1727)	Deutsches Historisches Museum, Berlin	Frans von Stampart (attributed to) (1675–1750)
	Nicholas Ferry, called Bébé, With Dog (c 1760)	Musée Historique Lorrain, Nancy	Anonymous (mid-18th century)
	Portrait of the Dwarf Count J. Boruwlaski, 1793–1837 (n.d.)	Museum Narodowe, Krakow, Poland	Unknown German painter
	Abendgesellschaft (Evening Gathering) (c 1847) (Self-portrait)	Staatliche Museen, Preussischer Kulturbesitz, Berlin	Adolph von Menzel (1815–1905)
• **Miscellaneous**			
◇ Mucopoly-saccharidosis (possibly)	*Christ Before Pilate* (c 1420)	Landesmuseum, Mainz	Master of the Oberstein Altar (active 1400–1420)
	The Dispute of St. Catherine (1525)	Boymans-van Beuningen Museum, Rotterdam	Jan Provoost (c 1465–1529)
◇ Other/various	*Charles Emmanuel I as a Child with his Court Dwarf* (before 1572)	Galleria Sabauda, Turin	Giacomo Vighi, called d'Argenta (c 1510–1573)
	Archduke Ferdinand with a Court Dwarf (1604) (hypothyroidism possibly)	Kunsthistorisches Museum, Vienna	Joseph Heintz the Elder (1564–1609)
	El Niño de Vallecas – Francisco Lezcano (1637) (hypothyroidism possibly)	Prado, Madrid	Velázquez (1599–1660)
	Dwarf with a Dog (1643)	Formerly Lederer Collection, Vienna	Jusepe de Ribera (1591–1652)
	Boys with Dwarfs (1646)	Stedelijk van Abbemuseum, Eindhoven	Jan Miense Molenaer (c 1610–1668)

110

DISORDER	PAINTING Title (date)	Location	ARTIST
	Jacoba Maria van Wassenaer or Bernardina Margriet van Raesfeld (1660)	Mauritshuis, The Hague	Jan Steen (c 1625–1679)
	Gregorio the Dwarf (1908)	Hermitage, St. Petersburg	Ignacio Zuloaga (1870–1945)
Epidermolysis bullosa	*Head of a Young Man* (early 16th century)	Fogg Art Museum, Cambridge, Massachusetts	Hans Holbein The Younger (1497/8–1543)
Epidermolysis bullosa (possibly syphilis)	*Heritage* (1899)	Munch Museum, Oslo	Edvard Munch (1863–1944)
Female hirsutism	*The Bearded Woman of Peñaranda* (c 1590s)	Prado, Madrid	Juan Sánchez Cotán (1561–1627)
	Magdalena Ventura (1631)	Lerma Foundation, Toledo	Jusepe de Ribera (1591–1652)
	Woman with a Beard (1957)	Private collection, UK	L. S. Lowry (1887–1976)
Hapsburg jaw	*Emperor Charles V at Mühlberg* (1547)	Prado, Madrid	Titian (c 1487–1576)
Hemiplegia (see also clubfoot)	*The Clubfooted Boy* (1642)	Louvre, Paris	Jusepe de Ribera (1591–1652)
Hypertrichosis universalis	*Portrait of Peter Gonzales and his Children* (c 1582)	Kunsthistorisches Museum, Vienna	Bavarian (Artist unknown)
Klippel-Feil anomaly	*Illustrations of the Book of Job* (1825)	—	William Blake (1757–1827)
Lesch-Nyhan syndrome (possibly)	*Three Miracles of Saint Zenobius* (c 1490–1510) (Zenobius exorcizes two young men gnawing their own flesh)	National Gallery, London	Sandro Botticelli (1445–1510)
Mental disease (epilepsy, madness, hysteria etc.)	*The Cure for Folly* (c 1480)	Prado, Madrid	Hieronymus Bosch (c 1450–1516)
	St. Catherine Exorcising a Possessed Woman (15th century)	Denver Art Museum, Denver, Colorado	Girolamo de Benvenuto (1470–c 1524)
	Healing of the Madman (c 1496)	Accademia, Venice	Vittore Carpaccio (c 1465–1526)
	The Cure of Folly (c 1556)	Prado, Madrid	Jan Sanders van Hemessen (c 1500–1575)
	The Extraction of the Stone (1650–1665)	Boymans-van Beuningen Museum, Rotterdam	Jan Steen (c 1626–1679)
	A Quack Drawing Stones from the Head of a Patient (Dutch school, 17th century)	Boymans-van Beuningen Museum, Rotterdam	Attributed to Jan de Bray (c 1627–1697)
	The Madhouse from The Rake's Progress (1734)	John Soane Museum, London	William Hogarth (1697–1764)
	The Madhouse of Saragossa (1794)	Meadows Museum, Dallas, Texas	Francisco Goya (1746–1828)
	The Madhouse (c 1800)	Academia San Fernando, Madrid	Francisco Goya (1746–1828)
	A Case of Mania (etching) (1838)	National Library of Medicine, Bethesda, Maryland	Ambroise Tardieu (1818–1879)
	Mania Succeeded by Dementia (etching) (1838)	Philadelphia Museum of Art	Ambroise Tardieu (1818–1879)
	Maniac During an Attack (etching) (1838)	Library, Faculty of Medicine, Paris	Jean Esquirol (1772–1840)
	The San Bonifacio Asylum (1865)	International Gallery of Modern Art, Venice	Telemaco Signorini (1835–1901)
	Electric Shock Treatment (1908)	Munch Museum, Oslo	Edvard Munch (1863–1944)
	Insane People at Mealtime (drypoint) (1914)	Philadelphia Museum of Art	Erich Heckel (1883–1970)
	The Psychiatrist (1945)	City Art Gallery, Birmingham	Stanley Spencer (1891–1959)
	Portrait of Dr Fritz Perls (1966)	Otto Dix Foundation, Vaduz, Liechtenstein	Otto Dix (1891–1969)
Noonan's syndrome (possibly)	*Among those Left* (1929)	Museum of Art, Carnegie Institute, Pittsburgh, Pennsylvania	Ivan Le Lorraine Albright (1897–1983)
Pectus carinatum	*Agosta the Pigeon-chested Man and Rasha the Black Dove* (1929)	Private Collection	Christian Schad (1894–1982)

DISORDER	PAINTING		ARTIST
	Title (date)	Location	
Phocomelia	*Girl with Wooden Leg and No Arms* (1514) (possibly gross trauma)	Public Art Museum, Basle	Urs Graf (c 1485–1527/28)
	Charles Emmanuel I of Savoy as a Child Accompanied by a Dwarf (1573)	National Gallery, Turin	Giacomo Vighi, called Argenta (c 1510–1573)
	Mother with Deformed Infant (c 1805)	Louvre, Paris	Francisco de Goya (1746–1828)
Prader-Willi syndrome (possibly)	*Eugenia Martinez Vallejo, La Monstrua* (c 1680)	Prado, Madrid	Juan Carreño de Miranda (1614–1685)
Pyknodysostosis	Various self-portraits	—	Henri de Toulouse-Lautrec (1864–1901)
Spastic paraplegia	*Child on all Fours (after Muybridge)* (1961)	Gemeentemuseum, The Hague	Francis Bacon (1909–1992)
Strabismus	Various self- and other portraits	—	Albrecht Dürer (1471–1528)
	Fedra Inghirami (1516)	Pitti, Florence	Raphael (1483–1520)
	Margrave Albrecht von Brandenburg, Duke of Prussia (1528)	Herzog Anton Ulrich Museum, Brunswick	Lucas Cranach (1472–1553)
	Portrait of Calabazas (c 1632)	Cleveland Museum of Art, Cleveland, Ohio	Velázquez (1599–1660)
	Archibald Campbell (c 1660)	National Portrait Gallery, Edinburgh	David Scougall (active 1654–1677)
	Little Girl with a Squint (c 1961)	Gracefield Art Centre, Dumfries	Joan Eardley (1921–1963)
Synophrys	Various self-portraits	Museum of Modern Art, New York & Private collections	Frida Kahlo (1907–1954)
Thoracopagus	*Joined Twins* (n.d.)	Gemeentemuseum, The Hague	E. C. van der Maas (1577–1656)
White forelock (possibly acquired)	*James McNeill Whistler* (1885)	Metropolitan Museum, New York	William Merritt Chase (1849–1916)
	James McNeill Whistler (c 1895)	Kupferstichkabinett, Berlin	Thomas R. Way (1861–1913)